W9-CKH-143

# THE GREAT LIFE MAKEOVER

# THE
# GREAT LIFE
# MAKEOVER

A Couples' Guide to

**WEIGHT, MOOD, and SEX**

for the Best Years of Your Life—

and Your Relationship

## DANIEL A. MONTI, MD, and
## ANTHONY J. BAZZAN, MD

with CAROL COLMAN

**COLLINS** LIVING
*An Imprint of HarperCollins Publishers*

THE GREAT LIFE MAKEOVER. Copyright © 2008 by DANIEL A. MONTI, MD, and ANTHONY J. BAZZAN, MD. All rights reserved. Printed in the United States of America. No part of this book may be used or reproduced in any manner whatsoever without written permission except in the case of brief quotations embodied in critical articles and review. For information, address HarperCollins Publishers, 10 East 53rd Street, New York, NY 10022.

HarperCollins books may be purchased for educational, business, or sales promotional use. For information, please write Special Markets Department, HarperCollins Publishers, 10 East 53rd Street, New York, NY 10022.

FIRST EDITION

*Designed by Susan Yang*

Library of Congress Cataloging-in-Publication Data has been applied for.

ISBN 978-0-06-143540-9

08   09   10   11   12   OV/RRD   10   9   8   7   6   5   4   3   2   1

# CONTENTS

INTRODUCTION ..... vii

**PART ONE**

## HOW'S YOUR SEX LIFE?

**CHAPTER ONE:** WHEN SEX STOPS FEELING GOOD FOR HER ..... 3

**CHAPTER TWO:** THE HARD TRUTH ABOUT SEX FOR HIM ..... 16

**PART TWO**

## FRAZZLED, FAT, AND FATIGUED

**CHAPTER THREE:** WHEN YOU'RE FEELING DOWN ..... 35

**CHAPTER FOUR:** THE LOWDOWN ON FAT ..... 46

**CHAPTER FIVE:** NOT GETTING ANY SLEEP . . .
FOR ALL THE WRONG REASONS ..... 64

**PART THREE**

## YOUR GREAT LIFE MAKEOVER

**CHAPTER SIX:** SEX MAKEOVER ..... 87

**CHAPTER SEVEN:** DIET MAKEOVER ..... 122

**CHAPTER EIGHT:** EXERCISE MAKEOVER ..... 154

2303

# CONTENTS

**CHAPTER NINE:** HORMONE MAKEOVER ..... 177

**CHAPTER TEN:** SUPPLEMENT MAKEOVER ..... 209

**CHAPTER ELEVEN:** MOOD MAKEOVER ..... 229

SELECTED BIBLIOGRAPHY ..... 241

INDEX ..... 249

# INTRODUCTION

**HER**

*Since menopause, Julie has been losing sleep and gaining weight. She was tired, cranky, and unhappy with herself, and sex was the last thing on her mind. But it seemed to Julie that sex was always first and foremost on her husband's mind. The tension between the couple had gotten so bad that they dreaded being alone together.*

**HIM**

*About a year ago, Alex, a 45-year-old accountant, started having difficulty getting an erection. Alex was so embarrassed by his problem that he no longer initiated sex with his wife, Kathy, and was unreceptive to her advances. Kathy became so cold and distant that Alex began to feel she was rejecting him. The couple had not had sex—or even a meaningful conversation—for nine months, and the lack of intimacy was taking its toll on their relationship.*

## THE THREE HOT-BUTTON ISSUES OF MIDLIFE: SEX, WEIGHT, AND MOOD

These stories are typical of those we hear from the men and women we see at the Jefferson-Myrna Brind Center of Integrative Medicine at Thomas Jefferson University and Hospital. Our patients seek our help because their lives are not the way they used to be . . . or the way they want them to be. Their sex lives are shot. They're gaining weight and getting flabbier. They're tired and stressed out. And they're determined to do something about it.

Until recently, many couples like these would have dismissed their sex problems with "What do you expect? We're middle aged." The new generation of midlife couples *expect* a great deal more. They expect to have great sex, great health, and a great life well into their later decades.

But despite a youthful mindset, real physical changes occur starting around age 40—and sometimes even younger—that can interfere with couples' enjoyment of life in the bedroom and elsewhere.

The three hot-button issues of midlife—*sex, weight,* and *mood*—come to a head at this time. And they can feed on one another, making a bad situation even worse.

- **SEX**

  A decline in the production of sex hormones can dampen libido and diminish sexual capacity in both women and men.

- **WEIGHT**

  A slowdown in metabolism makes it harder to maintain muscle and keep off excess fat. The inevitable weight gain can worsen hormonal problems.

- **MOOD**

  Chronically high levels of stress can aggravate midlife symptoms, accelerate aging, disrupt your hormones, make you fat and flabby, and put you in a very bad mood. Stress is certainly not conducive to good health, good sex, or good relationships.

To compound the problem, by midlife people are likely to be taking one or more prescription medications, such as beta-blockers for high blood pressure, or antidepressants for depression. These drugs often have sexual side effects, including lowering libido, making erections more difficult, and interfering with orgasm—not to mention that many disrupt sleep, and some can even cause weight gain.

Men and women are surprisingly clueless about what's going on with their partners—physically and emotionally—during midlife. It's difficult for a man to strike up a conversation with his wife or girlfriend and say, "Gee, honey, I'm not the stud I used to be. I just can't perform as well in bed, and I may need your help in this area." It's equally difficult for a woman to say to her husband or boyfriend, "This perimenopausal stuff is making me crazy. My body is changing, and sometimes sex hurts, and we need to change what we're doing."

Many people become so wrapped up in their own problems that they are often oblivious to the impact these problems could be having on their partners. This book provides couples with the information they need, along with clear guidelines on how to address these issues in a nonthreatening, hopeful, and helpful way.

The telltale physical and emotional changes of midlife can have a profound impact on a couple. Many patients are dragged in to see us by their spouses or partners. Desperate husbands and boyfriends seek help for wives and girlfriends who have lost their sex drive, are not enjoying sex the way they used to, or are being made miserable by menopause. Unhappy wives and girlfriends bring in husbands or boyfriends who are ignoring important symptoms that could lead to serious health problems (as men often do), can't perform the way they used to in bed, or are irritable and difficult to live with.

*Our goal is nothing less than a complete life makeover. We want you to have a great life, and we're going to show you how. Within the pages of this book, you will find the tools you need to get your health, your life, and your relationship back on track.*

## THE ANTI-GERIATRICIANS

Dr. Monti, the director of the Center, is a physician with a specialty in psychiatry, lifestyle coaching, and integrative health. Dr. Bazzan is a geriatrician and a specialist in aging. He is also our hormone specialist and heads the Andropause and Menopause Program at the Center. (Andropause, also known as male menopause, refers to the decline of testosterone and other changes that occur in midlife men.) We are the only geriatrician-psychiatrist team we know of to head a university-based program for both male and female menopause.

We sometimes call ourselves anti-geriatricians because we aim to keep our patients as youthful as possible for as long as possible. Our real interest is in helping our patients avoid the pitfalls of aging. We both had traditional medical school experiences. We were taught that the geriatrician's role was to manage the chronic diseases of aging with drugs and that it was nearly impossible to cure or prevent these diseases. Fortunately, there has been a seismic shift in belief about the role of the geriatrician. Today, we believe that we can do both. There is a new generation of doctors who are not interested in waiting to fix what's already broken. We're trying to prevent things from becoming broken in the first place.

Dr. Bazzan's job is to repair the "hardware" that runs the body—he makes sure that whatever systems are down are back in working order. Dr. Monti's job is to reinstall the "software" that programs the body; he teaches patients how to change the behaviors or lifestyle that may have been causing their problems in the first place.

We are both passionate believers in integrative medicine: We strive to correct the underlying problem causing the symptom so that the body can function the way it's supposed to, and we acknowledge that health is a confluence of all domains of life—mind, body, spirit, and community. And this is true whether we're treating sexual dysfunction, heart disease, diabetes, depression, or any other medical condition. We don't put a bandage over a problem and try to hide it. We try to fix it on as many levels as possible. And we integrate as many options into our treatment plans as is reasonable. We distinguish integrative medicine from alternative medicine, which implies an exclusion of conventional Western medicine. To the contrary, we are primarily guided by our medical training and all the emerging data from various realms of scientific research.

However, as practitioners of integrative medicine, we have a treatment arsenal that extends far beyond the usual pharmaceuticals. We embrace all scientifically validated therapies, including diet, exercise, and stress reduction. Although we use medication when necessary, much of what we recommend can be achieved without a prescription pad: We emphasize aggressive lifestyle intervention that readers can do on their own.

# REBALANCING HORMONES

As women reach menopause they experience a precipitous decline in sex hormone production. This can result in some very unpleasant symptoms, including hot flashes, vaginal dryness, decreased libido, moodiness, and weight gain.

Until recently, menopausal symptoms were routinely treated with synthetic hormones, but studies linking hormone replacement therapy (HRT) with an increased risk of cancer and other diseases have discouraged physicians from prescribing hormones. As a result, many women are forced to choose between two evils: being made miserable by their symptoms, or risking cancer. We offer women a third option—a combination of lifestyle changes, such as the right diet and exercise and a stress reduction program, which can be highly effective in terms of easing menopausal symptoms.

If lifestyle changes aren't sufficient, we consider HRT, but only after we carefully assess the benefits versus the risks.

We use the latest medical technology to screen out men and women who are at high risk of developing cancer and therefore should not be using hormones. We also closely monitor our patients who are taking hormones and show them how to minimize the cancer risk. Some people metabolize hormones poorly, breaking them down into toxic, potentially cancer-causing substances in their bodies. And that's true whether hormones are made by your own body or taken in the form of HRT. Fortunately, there are simple blood tests that can detect this problem, and there are ways to deal with it, which we will discuss in later chapters.

We want to make one thing clear: ***We are not cheerleaders for HRT.*** It is not appropriate for everyone, and we understand that many people are wary of it. Yet, we believe that when done correctly and thoughtfully, hormone replacement (or, as we more accurately call it, hormone rebalancing) can be an effective option for many men and women who need it.

## INTRODUCTION

### Men Suffer, Too

Men also experience a decline in the production of testosterone, the hormone that is essential for sex drive, erectile function, and generally feeling energetic and positive about life. (Although testosterone is known as a male hormone, women make it too, although in much smaller amounts than men.) If a man doesn't make enough testosterone, he won't be thinking about sex, let alone want to have sex. In some men, testosterone levels decline gradually, which usually doesn't cause a problem, but sometimes testosterone levels can fall precipitously. Low testosterone may be caused or aggravated by many factors, including genetics, poor diet (especially if it is high in animal fat), a sedentary lifestyle, and even chronic stress. In addition to making lifestyle changes, men with low testosterone levels often benefit from HRT, which in this case entails boosting testosterone back to normal. (We explain more about our HRT protocol for men and women in Chapter 9, "Hormone Makeover.")

### Beyond the Little Blue Pill

As men age, some may experience a decline in sex drive and also have difficulty getting or maintaining an erection. Judging by the constant barrage of commercials on television for erectile dysfunction (ED) drugs such as Viagra, Levitra, or Cialis, you would think that this problem can be solved by popping a pill. It's not so easy. Minor changes in sexual function are no cause for alarm. But if these problems are severe enough to inhibit sexual activity, they may not be within the normal scope of aging. They often indicate an underlying health issue such as hormonal deficiency, heart disease, diabetes, or even a psychological problem, any of which could be caused, if not aggravated, by lifestyle. Prescribing a drug to treat erectile dysfunction without a proper medical assessment may mask a symptom of a problem that needs treatment. That said, we sometimes do prescribe ED drugs, but again, this is a thoughtful process that requires an understanding of where you are physically and emotionally.

A recent study found that a third of men with ED who had been given prescriptions for an ED drug could not perform sexually after taking the first pill.

They were so disappointed that they gave up on sex completely. We try to avoid that kind of outcome.

Our aim is to restore overall sexual function—not just temporarily for a few hours or a weekend with the help of a pill—but for the rest of a man's life. And this is best done by addressing the underlying cause of the problem. Sometimes the right nutrition and exercise program can restore sexual function enough so that drugs are not needed.

*The Great Life Makeover* is divided into three sections:

- **Part I: How's Your Sex Life?** reviews the major sexual and physical issues facing men and women.
- **Part II: Frazzled, Fat, and Fatigued** examines the interrelationship between weight, lack of sleep, mood, and how it affects couples in and out of the bedroom.
- **Part III: Your Great Life Makeover** consists of the Sex Makeover, Diet Makeover, Exercise Makeover, Hormone Makeover, Supplement Makeover, and Mood Makeover.

## YOUR GREAT LIFE MAKEOVER

At the core of the book is the Great Life Makeover—our comprehensive lifestyle program geared for the midlife body, which addresses the three hot-button issues of midlife: sex, weight, and mood. Weight loss, increased physical activity, and stress reduction exercises can often boost the body's own production of hormones and reduce or even eliminate some of the unpleasant symptoms associated with both menopause and andropause.

### SEX MAKEOVER

Despite the fact that sex may now be possible, there is often residual friction between the couple that prevents them from having a satisfying sex life. We work with couples individually and together, helping them to reconnect on an emotional level so they can once again feel comfortable with physical intimacy—not just in bed but in all aspects of their relationship.

This part of the program shows you how to reboot your love life, reestablish intimacy, and reinvigorate your relationship. It provides specific language and techniques that enable you to approach difficult and sensitive issues with your partner without making him or her angry and defensive.

## DIET MAKEOVER

Our diet is an extraordinarily potent tool to restore health, energy, and sexual function in men and women. Within a short time, we see a dramatic improvement in hormone levels and cardiovascular risk factors (such as blood lipids and inflammatory markers). Try our diet for three weeks, and we guarantee you will feel better than you have in years.

## EXERCISE MAKEOVER

When it comes to dealing with sex, weight, and mood problems, regular exercise is one of the most effective—if not THE most effective—treatment for all three. We offer a quick, simple exercise program that you can do alone or with your partner.

## HORMONE MAKEOVER

You've undoubtedly heard lots of information—and misinformation—about hormones. Here we present the pros and cons of HRT and provide you with the facts that you (along with your doctor) need to make a smart decision. We believe that these decisions should be made on a case-by-case basis, weighing the risks versus the benefits, and based on a patient's family and medical history and lifestyle.

## SUPPLEMENT MAKEOVER

We believe that a good diet is critical for optimal health and that supplements can't compensate for poor nutrition. We do, however, recommend a select group of supplements that we believe can help rebalance hormones, help maintain normal metabolism, and preserve health.

## MOOD MAKEOVER

The role of stress is grossly underestimated in terms of its impact on your health, sex life, and relationships. The Mood Makeover will show you easy ways to de-stress your life and boost your mood. The daily routine of simple breathing and relaxation exercises will keep you calm and focused.

# WORK WITH YOUR PHYSICIAN

This book is intended to be a general guide: The information in it is the very same we give our patients during their extensive initial consultations. We hope to help you work with your doctor so that you, too, can benefit from a more comprehensive lifestyle approach to health management. Since many aspects of our program are designed to be implemented outside of our office, you too will be able to start making the changes we prescribe for many men and women in their middle years.

Start by making an appointment with your internist or family practitioner. Most of the procedures and tests discussed in this book can be performed by your regular physician. In rare cases, your physician may refer you to a specialist if you have a problem that requires special attention.

We wrote this book to make a difference. For years we have been helping men and women get a better grip on their health and their relationships, and thereby improve their quality of life.

Why couples? While we are glad to work with individuals and often do, our preference is to work with you AND your significant other. It is important that you understand and support each other in having a satisfying, more healthful, and more fulfilling life. Just as poor health behaviors are far reaching and affect the system on many levels, positive health behaviors do the same. Believe it or not, having a good relationship is a positive health behavior; in fact, research suggests that it might be the most important one! Your attitude, stress levels, and relationship can affect your health as much as your cholesterol levels—perhaps even more so.

Despite some of the hurdles that midlife couples must overcome, their relationships can be stronger than ever. One of the positive uplifting messages of *The Great Life Makeover* is that sex during midlife can be terrific as long as both partners are open and honest with each other. A young body may have the physical edge over a midlife body, but youth has its constraints. A mature couple who know each other well may be more at ease with each other and able to be exploratory in a way they may not have felt comfortable with twenty years ago.

As one of our patients recently put it, "Okay, I'm not 25 anymore. And I don't have the same libido as a 25-year-old, even with testosterone therapy. But there's something even better about our relationship now. I never really opened up to my wife before. I kept things to myself. We can really talk to each other now, and I feel closer to her. I'm looking forward to our future together."

# PART ONE

# HOW'S YOUR SEX LIFE?

## CHAPTER ONE

# WHEN SEX STOPS FEELING GOOD FOR HER

**HER**

*"He's got the libido of an 18-year-old, and I don't. Sometimes I feel dead below the waist, I try to get turned on, but nothing happens. And when we do have sex, it can hurt."*

**HIM**

*"She doesn't want to have sex as much as I do. But even when we do, she's not really enjoying it. I love her. I want things to be better."*

Nancy, an attractive 52-year-old artist, had been divorced for ten years before moving in with her fiancé, Robert, a very youthful 58. But what should have been a joyful time was marred by disagreements over sex. Specifically, he wanted it every day, and she didn't. For Nancy, having sex once or twice a week was more than enough. Even then, she had to really, really push herself before she felt sexually turned on. Sex wasn't always a struggle for Nancy. But like so many women in the midst of menopause, Nancy was experiencing physical and emotional changes that were making sex the last thing on her mind.

Nancy is not alone in finding that sex is not all it should be for women in midlife. A 2007 study of menopausal women revealed that 54% of the women surveyed reported a decrease in sexual activity after menopause. Almost half of all women said that they avoided sex because of physical discomfort. About three-quarters of the women surveyed were in committed relationships and believed that sex was important. What was particularly telling was that less than half of the women in the study were not satisfied with the amount of sex they were having.

We see this phenomenon among midlife women in our practice. They know that sex is important for a relationship, and they would love to be having sex more, but obviously they feel limited by their physical symptoms. And who can blame them? If sex causes more pain than pleasure, most women—or men for that matter—would want to opt out.

## SHE SUFFERS IN SILENCE

At one time, women who suffered from sexual symptoms caused by menopause found an easy solution in HRT. Love it or hate it, HRT—yes, even those synthetic hormones we don't like—worked well for many women in terms of preserving sexual function. But now that HRT has fallen into disrepute, many women—and even their doctors—feel that women have no choice but to suffer through these symptoms. That's assuming that women even talk to their doctors about intimate issues; several studies suggest that they avoid potentially embarrassing topics. And so do their doctors.

Despite its bad rep, hormone replacement is still a viable treatment for women who are suffering during menopause or who want to avoid the symptoms associated with hormone depletion. We describe bioequivalent hormones for both women and men in Chapter 9, "Hormone Makeover," and we talk about the non-hormonal and over-the-counter solutions in Chapter 6, "Sex Makeover."

This begs the question, what is a "normal" menopause versus one that requires treatment? Insomnia, hot flashes, and mood swings are all normal symptoms; yet, they can affect women very differently depending on their lifestyles. For example, a woman who gets up early every morning to get to work will be more upset about losing sleep than another woman who works at home and can nap during the day. A woman who has low libido will be more concerned about her lack of sex drive if she has a partner who is very amorous than a woman who is alone or is with a man who is not all that interested. To a large extent, menopause is a subjective experience.

In comparison with men, women find that the transition to midlife is much more complicated. Most midlife men experience a gradual decline in the production of their primary hormone, testosterone. For some men, the drop in testosterone is so gradual that they hardly know it's happening. A healthy man can often stave off many of the physical changes that have become associated with aging, including ED and loss of libido. And if these problems do occur, they're usually not that difficult to fix.

Women, however, are another story. Perimenopause, the years leading up to menopause, and menopause itself (the cessation of menstruation), cause many physical and emotional changes that can put a strain on a couple's relationship.

The drop in the two hormones that regulate the menstrual cycle, progesterone and estrogen, can be quite abrupt and erratic. At the same time, women are also losing testosterone, which, as you will see, is as vital for their health and well-being as it is for men. These fluctuations in hormones can make a woman feel miserable. Furthermore, the anatomical changes that occur after menopause can make sex uncomfortable, if not painful.

Some lucky women sail through these years without experiencing significant discomfort. And many women discover that over time, as their bodies adjust to their new postmenopausal state, the symptoms that were driving them crazy disappear. Free from the fear of pregnancy and from the duties of raising children, some midlife women say they feel happier and sexier than ever once their hormones settle down. But many women need some additional help to navigate through these years.

## WHAT HAPPENS DURING MENOPAUSE?

In the not too distant past, menopause coincided with what we would call old age. At the turn of the past century, the average woman didn't make it past 50. Today, the average woman lives many decades beyond menopause and wants to live those years in a healthy, vital body with a sharp, active mind. But that's not what nature intended for women.

Women may not like to think of themselves solely in terms of their reproductive role, but nature views it differently. Women's bodies are designed to maintain optimal health throughout the childbearing years. Once women move out of their prime reproductive years, their body systems begin to wear down one by one. This is true for both men and women, but since women are the ones who the bear the children, they are hit harder.

The average age of menopause for women in the United States is 54, but hormone production begins to fall off long before, typically causing menstrual irregularities and other perimenopausal symptoms. In fact, many of the symptoms we associate with menopause, such as insomnia, hot flashes, and irritability, often begin during perimenopause.

For women, the decline in reproductive ability begins in their mid to late 30s and accelerates throughout the 40s. That's why, for every year over 30, it becomes increasingly difficult to get pregnant. Menopause is defined as the cessation of the menstrual cycle, which is caused by the depletion of living, viable eggs inside the ovaries. If you're a woman over 50 and you haven't had a period within one year, you are officially considered to be menopausal.

A girl is born with roughly half a million immature eggs, or follicles, in her ovaries; the monthly menstrual cycle revolves around preparing one of those eggs for a potential pregnancy. The cycle is usually divided into two parts: the estrogen phase and the progesterone phase. In the first part of the menstrual cycle (the estrogen phase), the pituitary releases follicle-stimulating hormone (FSH), which prepares one of the eggs for fertilization. The developing egg releases high amounts of estrogen, which brings about a drop in FSH production.

Women make three types of estrogens: estradiol, estrone, and estriol. Estradiol is the primary and most potent estrogen. It is responsible for normal menstrual flow and bone mineral density as well as mood, sex drive, proper function of the heart and blood vessels, skin elasticity, and brain and thyroid function. In other words, the influence of estrogen extends far beyond the reproductive system.

At about day 14, or mid cycle (the progesterone phase), there is a surge of luteinizing hormone (LH), which causes the egg to rupture, signaling to the ovaries to release the mature egg (now called the corpus luteum) into the fallopian tubes, where it travels to the uterus. The corpus luteum begins producing progesterone along with estrogen. The uterine lining thickens to support a possible pregnancy. If the egg is not fertilized, hormone levels drop, and the uterine lining is shed during the next menstrual period.

## Hormonal Ups and Downs

The egg is the "brain" that regulates the balance of hormones during the menstrual cycle. Once the supply of eggs dries up, hormone production sharply declines, creating an imbalance. The pituitary gland still produces FSH in a last-ditch effort to stimulate ovulation, but to no avail. Rising FSH levels are a sign that the ovaries are not producing enough estrogen. There are hormone fluctuations that can make women feel miserable, triggering hot flashes and night sweats.

Progesterone is the first hormone to go, falling steeply during perimenopause. By the time menopause is complete, a woman can lose up to 90% of this hormone. Progesterone can have a big impact on a woman's quality of life. As women lose progesterone they often experience problems sleeping and may feel anxious and more irritable.

Estrogen levels also begin to drop, albeit more slowly than progesterone, and

7

by the time a woman is menopausal, she has lost between 40% and 60% of her estrogen.

During this time, women lose another important hormone that has a profound impact on their lives, although it is not involved in the menstrual cycle. The production of testosterone drops by up to 90% in women. Similarly to progesterone, testosterone is important for mood, but it's also important for sex drive, body composition, bone density, and maintaining an overall feeling of well-being. For some women, the loss of testosterone is as bad as, if not worse than, the loss of estrogen.

It's important to remember that menopause is a process that plays out over time. For some women, the hormonal ups and downs can last a decade or longer, punctuated by difficult menstrual cycles. Some women may get their periods every three weeks; others may miss several periods and have a period only every few months or so in the years leading up to menopause. Our point is this: even while you're still menstruating you can still have miserable perimenopausal symptoms.

## The Vulnerable Periods

For many women, what we consider "aging" is accelerated after menopause. The first five years following menopause in particular are often the roughest in terms of a woman's health and well-being. The loss of hormones can make you feel miserable. Under ideal conditions, the adrenal glands should pick up the slack and produce some sex hormones; for many women, this does the trick. Very often, the adrenals don't produce enough of all three hormones to relieve symptoms or make a woman feel like herself again. This is particularly true for women who are under a great deal of stress (see Chapter 3, "When You're Feeling Down"). Learning how to de-stress can be an important step in relieving menopausal symptoms, and for that, we refer you to Chapter 11, "Mood Makeover."

Here's a rundown of the physical changes you are likely to experience as you reach menopause. Not all women experience all these changes at once, some may be hard hit, and some may breeze through them with very little difficulty.

## VAGINAL THINNING

The vaginal walls get thinner, which can make sexual intercourse painful. At the same time, there is a reduction in vaginal lubricant, the slippery coating produced by the Bartholin glands at the entrance of the vagina when a woman is aroused. Some women find that after menopause it takes longer to get aroused and to lubricate. They may be capable of making enough lubricant, but they need longer foreplay. Without lubricant, the friction created by the penis rubbing up against the vagina can be very irritating. The combination of vaginal thinning and loss of lubrication can make a woman feel negative about having sex. Furthermore, severe vaginal dryness can cause a sensation of burning and irritation that can be quite annoying.

These vaginal changes also make a woman more prone to bacterial and yeast infections, as well as urinary tract infections, which just add to her general discomfort.

Women with autoimmune diseases, such as lupus and rheumatoid arthritis, may have even more difficulty with lubrication than do women who do not have these diseases.

The solution to vaginal changes is not to have less sex—but more sex. Regular sexual activity can help keep the vaginal walls stronger and more flexible. Sex is also good for a couple's relationship and overall well-being. Having said this, we realize that it's important to first correct the problems that create sexual discomfort for women. We urge any woman with these problems to read Chapter 6, "Sex Makeover," and Chapter 9, "Hormone Makeover," to learn about things she can do on her own or with the help of her doctor.

## SKIN CHANGES

The skin is the body's largest organ and the one that is most noticeable. After menopause, there is a change in skin tone and texture, which can be quite dramatic. A woman's skin gets thinner, dryer, and more prone to wrinkles. Skin changes are primarily due to estrogen loss, which keeps the skin plumped up and supple. Lifestyle plays a major role, too. Women who have spent years in the sun without skin protection may wrinkle faster than others. Furthermore, women who smoke tend to look up to a decade older than do nonsmokers.

## BONE AND MUSCLE

About half of all women over 65 have osteoporosis, the thinning or wearing away of bone. After age 30, both men and women lose about 1% of their bone mass every year. Bone loss is significantly accelerated after menopause; the average woman loses 2% to 4% of her bone mass over the next decade. The postmenopausal bone loss is due to the drop in levels of both estrogen and testosterone. At the same time, there is a decline in muscle mass and muscle strength—a condition known as sarcopenia. These changes in both muscle and bone can be slowed down by regular weight-bearing exercise. HRT is probably the most effective way to stop and reverse bone loss for someone with diminished hormone levels.

Many women also complain of feeling "achy" in their muscles and joints, and this, too, is due to the loss of estrogen and testosterone.

## MEMORY AND MOOD

Midlife women often complain that they're not as sharp as they used to be, they can't remember things anymore, and they fear that they're "losing it." The good news, according to recent research, is that the so-called loss of mental function during midlife is not due to menopause. In other words, it is not inevitable. Now for the bad news: If you are suffering from cognitive problems, it could be a sign that you are under too much stress.

We've known for some time that estrogen plays a role in learning and memory, so it's been assumed that the decline in estrogen must trigger these changes in brain function. But when researchers recently tested the estrogen hypothesis on three groups of women: premenopausal, menopausal, and postmenopausal, it didn't pan out. Two noted neuropsychologists followed 800 women for six years, giving them a series of annual tests to monitor brain function. Surprisingly, they did not find a significant decline in brain function among the women as they moved through the stages of menopause—in fact, most of the test scores actually increased. Their conclusion was that estrogen loss due to menopause does not negatively alter brain function.

So what is behind these cognitive changes experienced by so many women? At least one major study has suggested that despite the hype, these changes in brain function are little more than urban legends—much talked about but not real. Another study, however, conducted by researchers at the University of Rochester, came up with a more plausible answer. As with previous studies, they did not find specific memory problems in women approaching menopause. When they probed further, however, they found that midlife women often had more difficulty "encoding," or learning new information. Although a woman may perceive this as a memory problem, in reality it isn't. Here's where it gets interesting—the researchers observed that menopausal women presented with a new mental challenge were responding the way people classically behave when they are under a great deal of stress. They cited the example of a patient being told that she is seriously ill by her doctor, and then not remembering the details of the conversation when she gets home. It's not that the patient can't remember what the doctor said; the reality is that she never really absorbed what he was saying because she was so upset.

Midlife can be a very stressful time for women, who not only are coping with physical and emotional changes but also may have to juggle work, child rearing, and caring for older relatives. With so much on their minds, it's no wonder that women may misplace their keys now and then, or blank out on someone's name.

Getting a handle on stress and maintaining a good nutritional status is critical to maintaining good brain function as well as good health. We provide specific tips on how to de-stress your brain and your body in Chapter 11, "Mood Makeover," and how to make sure it is getting the adequate fuel in Chapter 7, "Diet Makeover."

## THE LAST THING ON HER MIND

Many couples fall out of synch sexually during midlife, with men typically showing more interest in sex than women, though this is not always the case. From adolescence on, it's typically easier for men to get turned on than it is for women. For many guys, an available partner and a sexy magazine or movie do the trick. It's not surprising that this continues to be the case in midlife. And given all the changes that occur in women during this transition, it's not surprising that some women may go through times when they're simply not interested in sex. The disparity in sexual desire becomes a problem, however, if it creates tension within the relationship.

We've come a long way from the days when sex was associated primarily with reproduction. The sexual revolution of the mid-twentieth century brought about sweeping changes in our attitudes toward sex. We no longer view sex solely as the means to bear children; it is now considered an important bond between a couple that can enhance a relationship. From a biological point of view, however, our personal fulfillment is unimportant. Nature's primary concern is that we pass on our genes to future generations. Once we've completed this task, nature turns its attention elsewhere. Of course, we feel quite differently! We want those later years to be interesting and meaningful! They can be, and we can help you achieve that. As men and women live longer and have longer marriages, or take up with new partners later in life, today they expect that intimacy is part of the package.

Since the spectacular success of ED drugs, pharmaceutical companies have been racing to market the first drug for women to rev up sex drive. In fact, Viagra was even tested on women to see if it had any effect on libido; although the drug improved blood flow to the vagina, it did nothing to boost libido.

Female sex drive is a complex issue, and the solution is not as simple as correcting most cases of ED, which are typically caused by poor blood flow. Not so for libido. For women in particular, sex drive is dependent on many factors: some physical, some emotional.

One of the primary physical causes of low libido is fairly easy to fix. We have found—and studies confirm our findings—that women with abnormally low testosterone levels often have low libido. Once testosterone levels are brought back to normal, there is a marked increase in energy, mood, and sex drive.

But not every woman suffering from low libido is low in testosterone. Some women may actually want to have sex but are so physically uncomfortable that they are willing to forego it. In many cases, their partners are unaware of their physical discomfort and may be doing things during sex that exacerbate it. For example, menopausal women often need more foreplay, and they may find that some positions they used to like are now painful. This may sound simple, but if a couple has been making love for years the same way, and it's worked for them in the past, it may be difficult for one or both of them to accept that they need to change their routine. On the bright side, rediscovering each other can be very exciting and breathe new life into a relationship.

## Difficulty Achieving Orgasm

When a woman becomes sexually aroused, her heart beats faster and blood flow is directed to the pelvic area, causing the labia to swell or become engorged. Lack of estrogen can reduce blood flow, which can interfere with a woman's ability to become aroused. If a woman has poor circulation due to coronary artery disease or diabetes, engorgement can be affected. For both men and women, sexual intercourse ideally culminates with an orgasm, when the muscles in the pelvis contract rhythmically, producing feelings of pleasure. For women, an orgasm is dependent on the stimulation of the clitoris, a small organ on the upper part of the vulva of the vagina. The drop in estrogen and its subsequent effect on nerve function can hamper a woman's ability to have an orgasm, or can make orgasms less intense than in the past.

Women with high blood pressure are particularly prone to problems with lubrication and reaching orgasm; in part, this can be caused by medications that lower blood pressure.

Some menopausal women experience delayed orgasm: it takes longer for their clitoris to respond to stimulation, and some women may have difficulty reaching orgasm at all. Once again, the decline in estrogen and testosterone, weak pelvic floor muscles, vaginal thinning, and poor blood flow can interfere with the ability to have an orgasm, or with the quality of the orgasm. Numerous medications— including antidepressants—can also inhibit or delay orgasm. Similar to men, for women good health goes hand in hand with good sex. Even before they reach menopause, women with diabetes can have sexual problems, including lack of lubrication and orgasm difficulties.

## IT COMES BACK TO LIFESTYLE

A healthful lifestyle can also make a huge difference in how a woman looks and feels during the years leading up to menopause and afterward. Maintaining a normal weight through diet and exercise is critical for both physical and emotional health. Feeling attractive about her physical appearance is important for a woman's self-esteem. Furthermore, midlife weight increases a woman's risk for the development of heart disease, high blood pressure, diabetes, and arthritis, which are often treated with medication that can cause sexual side effects.

Many prescription drugs can interfere with a woman's sexual function. Some can inhibit arousal; others can prevent lubrication or delay orgasm—problems that are common during menopause. Antidepressants and medications to lower blood pressure are high on the list of sex-busting drugs. Common over-the-counter drugs, like antihistamines to treat your allergy symptoms, not only dry up your nose but may cause vaginal dryness as well. If a woman is considering taking any medication, she should talk to her doctor about the sexual side effects. Often you don't know how you react to a drug until you actually take it, so if you notice a change in either sex drive or function, talk to your doctor about switching to another drug.

## TOP SEX-BUSTING PRESCRIPTION DRUGS FOR WOMEN

### Antidepressants

**SSRI**

*fluoxetine* (Prozac), *paroxetine* (Paxil), *sertraline* (Zoloft)

**TRICYCLIC**

*amitriptyline* (Elavil), *nortriptyline* (Pamelor)

## Antihypertensives to Lower Blood Pressure

**ACE INHIBITORS**

*benazepril* (Lotensin), *captopril* (Capoten), *enalapril* (Vasotec), *quinapril* (Accupril), *ramipril* (Altace)

**ALPHA-INHIBITORS**

*prazosin* (Minipress), *doxazosin* (Cardura)

**BETA-BLOCKERS**

*propranolol* (Inderal), *carvedilol* (Coreg), *metoprolol succinate* (Toprol XL), *atenolol* (Tenormin), *metoprolol* (Lopressor)

**CALCIUM CHANNEL BLOCKERS**

*diltiazem* (Cardizem), *nifedipine* (Procardia), *verapamil* (Calan), *felodipine* (Plendil)

## GI-Ulcer Drugs

**H2 ANTAGONISTS**

*cimetidine* (Tagamet), *ranitidine* (Zantac)

## Painkillers

**OPIOIDS**

*hydromorphone* (Dilaudid), *oxycodone* (Percodan), *fentanyl* (Fentora)

CHAPTER TWO

# THE HARD TRUTH ABOUT SEX FOR HIM

**HIM**

*"The first few times it happened, I thought that it was one of those things that just happens to guys in their 50s. But when I had erection problems every time I tried to have sex, I could see that Lisa was getting worried about me. But I didn't want to talk about it."*

**HER**

*"We'd be watching the commercials on TV for Viagra, and I'd be dying to say something, but I didn't for quite a while. But I knew that erection problems could be a sign of a health problem. Not to mention the fact that I missed sex! So I finally had to say something. I think Steve was actually relieved when I did."*

It can happen to the best of guys, and the best of couples. According to the 1994 groundbreaking Massachusetts Male Aging Study, about 40% of all men at age 40 have some form of erectile dysfunction (ED). By age 70, about 70% of all men are affected by ED.

The textbook definition of erectile dysfunction is the inability to get or sustain an erection long enough to complete sexual intercourse, but there are degrees of this condition. Some men can't get hard at all; some men can't maintain enough rigidity to complete intercourse. Some men can maintain an erection only when they masturbate but not when they attempt intercourse. And some men have erections in the morning, when their levels of testosterone are at their highest, but have problems later in the day.

The normal physical changes that occur in men and women during midlife can affect their sex lives. As men age they are often not as sexually responsive as they were when they were younger. Men who used to fantasize about sex a lot may find that they hardly ever think about it. They may not get as hard as fast, or stay as hard as they used to. A guy who used to have an erection at the sight (or mere thought) of a pretty girl may now need more help from his partner in terms of manual or oral stimulation or other aids. Couples need to understand the physical changes that their partners are experiencing, and try to accommodate each other's needs. This has as much to do with good communication as having a good sexual technique. We talk more about this in Chapter 6, "Sex Makeover."

So when does ED officially become a problem? The rule of thumb is this: if a man can't sustain an erection long enough to complete sexual intercourse, and this has occurred more often than not over a six-month period, it is no longer considered within the range of normal. It's often a sign of an underlying physical or emotional problem—and very often it can quickly become a combination of both.

ED is not to be confused with premature ejaculation—that's when a man has no trouble getting an erection but reaches orgasm too quickly. This usually occurs in younger men and is more likely due to poor sexual technique than to poor health.

## MEN DON'T TELL; DOCS DON'T ASK

Since the debut of drugs for ED such as Viagra in 1998, and Cialis and Levitra later, the barrage of TV commercials for these products has made it somewhat easier for men to raise the topic with their doctors. Still, studies have shown that men typically don't tell their doctors about sexual problems, and many doctors don't ask. This is especially true for men (and women) over the age of 50. In a survey of 1,455 men ages 57 to 85 published in 2007 in the *New England Journal of Medicine*, only 38% of the men said they had talked about their sexual health with their doctors since they had turned 50. That's precisely the time when men and their physicians should be addressing these issues.

Let's face it: many men are still uncomfortable talking about their health in general and their sexual health in particular. Some doctors may be reluctant to bring it up because they fear embarrassing their patients . . . or themselves!

When a man doesn't feel as sexually charged as he once did, or can't perform the way he used to, it hits him where it hurts the most—his self-esteem. Men fear that they are losing their virility, the very essence of what makes them male.

So it's understandable that rather than embarrass her husband, Steve, Lisa kept quiet about their waning sex life. But Lisa and Steve had been together nearly twenty years, so it wasn't the dry spell in their sex life that worried Lisa. She was concerned that Steve's overall health seemed to be going steadily downhill. The usual energetic, upbeat man was so exhausted at the end of the day that when he came home, he crashed on the sofa for the night. Too tired to go the gym, Steven stopped working out and was putting on weight.

Lisa finally decided that she couldn't keep quiet any longer and insisted that Steve come to us for a checkup. By this point, Steve was so alarmed by how he felt that he reluctantly agreed to see us. It was a good thing, too. We gave Steve a complete physical examination, including a careful medical history, as well as laboratory tests to check blood lipids, blood sugar levels, hormone levels, and other important aspects of blood chemistry. It's very important that a doctor not dismiss ED as part of normal aging. It could also be a symptom of any number of possible problems, including cardiovascular disease, enlarged prostate, anemia, diabetes, kidney disease, liver disease, cancer, or neurological problems. It could also be a result of chronic alcoholism or drug abuse. We're not telling you this to frighten you, but you need to understand the importance of having a thorough physical exam to rule out any of these possibilities.

## The Prediabetes Connection

Our ED workup of Steve revealed something that is unfortunately all too common. He had metabolic syndrome, a condition characterized by a cluster of symptoms, including high blood sugar, high blood pressure, and high levels of bad cholesterol. Metabolic syndrome is sometimes called prediabetes because it often leads to Type 2 diabetes, also known as adult-onset diabetes. There are two types of diabetes: Type 1, formerly called juvenile diabetes, is caused by a failure of the pancreas to produce enough insulin, the hormone that controls blood sugar. Type 1 is usually a genetic problem that strikes early in life.

In contrast, Type 2 diabetes is a disease of lifestyle, and it is becoming an epidemic in this country. About 40% of all U.S. adults over 40 have prediabetes signs and symptoms. It is typically the result of a diet too high in sugary, processed foods and saturated fats—the typical American diet—and too little activity to burn it off.

In prediabetes, the pancreas pumps out high amounts of insulin in response to high levels of blood sugar. Under normal conditions, insulin should restore blood sugar back to normal, but the constant insulin surges have just the opposite effect. The cells of the body no longer respond to insulin effectively, leaving us with the worst of both worlds: elevated blood sugar levels AND elevated insulin, both of which cause problems.

High insulin is a double whammy for weight, as it works synergistically with bad diet to cause increased fat stores in the body. It doesn't just make you fat; it can be lethal. The resulting prediabetes is a major risk factor for cardiovascular disease and stroke.

Fortunately, metabolic syndrome can often be reversed before it develops into diabetes by making lifestyle changes recommended in the Diet and Exercise Makeovers. In some cases, medication and supplements to control blood sugar are also necessary, as in Steve's case.

We also found, as we often do in these cases, that Steve's testosterone level was lower than normal. We prescribed AndroGel, a topical testosterone gel that Steve rubbed into his skin twice a day. We also saw from his lab results that his body was making a little too much estrogen, which is not uncommon with andropausal men, especially those who have too much body fat. So we gave him some supplements to minimize the testosterone-to-estrogen conversion process and emphasized the importance of eating plenty of cruciferous vegetables, such as broccoli and cabbage, which help normalize hormones.

Within a few months, Steve's energy was restored and his health was back on track. Happily, the couple was able to resume their sex life, with the help of some counseling. As we discuss in Chapter 6, "Sex Makeover," once a couple has a problem, it can create anxiety that lingers even when the problem is resolved. Our success stories don't typically end with the couple eager to jump in the sack—more often they end with the couple ready to start talking to each other again about sex. The actual act of sex may occur weeks or months later, but when it does, the couple is physically and emotionally prepared.

The moral of this story is, don't ignore ED.

## GETTING TO THE CAUSE OF ED

ED is often an early symptom of many medical problems, especially heart disease. A 2006 article in the *European Heart Journal* found that ED can manifest itself two to three years before the onset of coronary artery disease, a primary cause of heart attack and stroke. To understand why, you need to know a bit about the mechanics of an erection.

When a man is sexually aroused, his brain sends a signal to the muscles in his penis to relax so that blood can flow to his penis, specifically into the blood vessels and spongy tissue called the corpus cavernosum or corpus spongiosum. This makes the penis hard, thus causing the erection.

But first things first. An erection is not likely to happen if a man is not aroused, and the ability to feel sexually charged is largely dependent on testosterone, the hormone that regulates sex drive. If a man doesn't have enough testosterone, even if he can get an erection for sex, he may not be very interested.

Or if a man is very stressed out, or anxious about having an erection (which can happen after a bout of ED), that can also interfere with his ability to have an erection.

Similarly, if there is nerve damage, this can prevent the signals from the brain from being transmitted via the spinal cord to the penis, telling it that he's interested in having sex. Nerve damage can be caused by a spinal cord injury, a stroke, or even diabetes. After prostate surgery, it is not unusual for a man to experience erectile problems.

An erection is also dependent on good circulation. If blood flow is impaired in any way, it can interfere with the ability to get or sustain the erection. And here's where cardiovascular health comes into play. The arteries delivering blood to the penis are smaller than the coronary arteries delivering blood to the heart. This means that if a man is prone to developing atherosclerosis or clogged arteries, it is likely to strike the smaller arteries first because they will become narrow faster, thus blocking blood flow. That's why erection problems are often the precursor of heart problems.

Treatment of the root causes of the heart disease is often the first step in treating ED. Bringing high blood lipids back to normal (lowering elevated LDL cholesterol, or high triglycerides) and reducing high blood pressure can help reverse damage to the arteries, and that will improve blood flow.

Medication is not our first line of defense. Losing weight can help improve blood lipids, especially if you are following the right diet. Regular exercise and weight loss can help lower blood pressure. As a side benefit, weight loss and exercise will also help normalize hormone levels. And while you're cleaning up your act, you're also feeling a lot better, which will make you want to have sex now that you're able to do so.

Below, we review our comprehensive approach for sexual dysfunction in men. We provide this information so you can work with your doctor to help regain your health as well as improve your sex life.

## In the Doctor's Office

First, we screen for any common medical conditions that could be interfering with libido and erectile function, such as hormonal imbalances, diabetes, heart disease, neurological disease, or depression. We ask our patients to fill out detailed questionnaires on their medical history and lifestyle, and we follow up with a complete physical examination. You'd be surprised how many patients hold back vital information because they believe it's not relevant, they're embarrassed by it, or they're afraid that it's a sign of something serious. It's important to be honest with your doctor and tell him or her about any symptoms you may be experiencing, sexual or otherwise. Your input can help your doctor make the correct diagnosis.

We also understand that in this era of managed care, many patients feel that their doctors are in a hurry and don't allow enough time for the patient interview. Unfortunately, this is a reality of modern life, and it's not likely to change. You can make the best use of your doctor's time by bringing a written list of your symptoms to refer to during the patient interview. It's also wise to write down any medications you are taking, including supplements.

## Hormone Level Check

When a man complains of low sex drive, fatigue, and "not feeling like myself anymore," one of the first things we do is check his hormone levels. More often than not, these men are deficient in testosterone. Testosterone is not just important for libido but is essential for the maintenance of muscle and bone. Men who are deficient in testosterone can work out to the point of exhaustion and still have nothing to show for it but flab.

Although testosterone is associated with "aggressive" behavior, in reality, psychological studies show that men who are low in testosterone are often angrier and more irritable than men with normal levels. Men with low testosterone are also more likely to be depressed.

Testosterone is primarily made in the testes, but a small amount is also made in the adrenal glands. Luteinizing hormone (LH) and follicle-stimulating hormone (FSH), made by the anterior pituitary, regulate its metabolism. LH controls the production and secretion of testosterone by the Leydig cells of the testes, and FSH stimulates the production of sperm. Testosterone is known as an androgen, or male hormone, but it is also found in both sexes. (Women make testosterone in the ovaries and adrenal glands.)

Men make more testosterone than women—an adult male produces twenty to thirty times the amount of testosterone as does an adult woman—because it is vital for male sexual development. Testosterone is the hormone that turns boys into men. Once puberty hits, rising testosterone levels cause the penis and testicles to grow and mature, the voice to deepen, body hair to grow, and muscles and bone to develop. Testosterone revs up libido and sexual desire and is crucial for the formation of sperm. A byproduct of testosterone, dihydrotestosterone, is one factor that helps produce an erection. Although testosterone is usually not the critical factor in ED, if a man doesn't have enough of this hormone, he's not going to be very interested in sex to begin with, and his fertility may also be impaired.

### He Makes Estrogen, Too

Just as women make testosterone, men make estrogen, albeit in minute quantities. The correct testosterone-to-estrogen balance must be maintained or a man will begin to lose some of his masculine features. As men age, some of their testosterone may be converted by fat cells into estradiol, a type of estrogen, which itself can have a byproduct that can increase the risk of prostate cancer. The more fat cells a man has—especially abdominal fat—the higher the risk of producing too much estrogen.

Men who are low in testosterone may experience negative changes in body composition, specifically less muscle and more fat, a loss of body hair, and in some the development of gynecomastia (enlarged male breasts), a sign of excess estrogen.

There are several ways to measure testosterone: total testosterone, free testosterone, and a protein called sex-hormone-binding globulin, or SHBG. Most of the testosterone in the body is bound to SHBG and is released into the bloodstream as it is needed. Only a very small amount of total testosterone in the body is free testosterone, that is, unbound and available for use by our cells and tissues. With age, the amount of testosterone attached to SHBG increases, leaving less testosterone for use. If you only measure total testosterone, you may get a false impression of how much testosterone is actually available. We have often seen men with normal total testosterone levels but high SHBG and deficient-free testosterone.

Despite the fact that many of the men we see have had obvious symptoms of testosterone deficiency—fatigue, loss of libido, poor muscle mass—their primary physicians failed to check their hormone levels. *If you suspect that you are low in testosterone, be sure to ask your doctor to perform this test.* We routinely order a hormone panel to check for low testosterone and elevated estrogen, both of which could interfere with sex drive and sexual function. In a man, a high level of estrogen is a sign that he is converting the little testosterone he has left into estrogen. If a man is overweight, chances are he's making the excess estrogen because his fat cells are secreting aromatase, an enzyme that converts testosterone into estrogen. Whatever the reason, his tissues are suffering from the effect of too much estrogen and too little testosterone.

## Thyroid Problems: Rare But Often Overlooked

By far the most common endocrine disorder causing ED is low testosterone, but in rare cases thyroid dysfunction can affect the male reproductive system.

Hyperthyroidism (excess production of thyroid hormone) has been associated with an increase in total serum testosterone levels but also with increased SHBG levels. The increase in SHBG causes a relative decrease in the free testosterone levels, so you can have high total testosterone but low free testosterone, which doesn't do you much good.

In severe cases, there is an elevation of the serum LH (negative feedback), a further increase in serum testosterone, and an increase in serum estradiol. As a result of the increase in circulating estrogens, these men with hyperthyroidism may have gynecomastia (enlarged breasts), spider angiomas (a group of small blood vessels that are close to the surface of the skin), and a decrease in libido. Treatment of the hyperthyroidism reverses the symptoms and signs of the disorder. In hypothyroidism, LH and FSH are usually elevated, the serum testosterone and SHBG are usually low, and the free testosterone can be either increased, decreased, or normal.

Some men with hypothyroidism (low thyroid hormone production) may complain of ED; in this setting, replacement with thyroxin (thyroid hormone) rarely improves potency on its own. Testosterone replacement may also be necessary. *(If we suspect thyroid hormone imbalance, we may do further testing before prescribing treatment. See "His Hormone Makeover" on page 201.)*

In addition to the standard laboratory tests for hormone levels, dyslipidemia (bad blood fats), and abnormal blood sugar levels, we check for other markers that may reveal important information about a man's health and possible causes of his sexual problems.

## Inflammatory Factors

We check for levels of key inflammatory factors, such C-reactive protein, IL–6, LP-PLA2, and PA-I, which can be very revealing in terms of assessing current health and the risk of developing a serious disease down the road. Inflammation is a contributing factor in virtually every chronic illness, especially in heart disease, obesity, and diabetes, the prime medical causes of erectile dysfunction. The highly inflammatory, overly processed diet consumed by most Americans is the prime reason why these diseases are rampant in this country. Understanding the connection between elevated inflammatory factors and difficulty in the bedroom can be very persuasive in terms of convincing a man it's time to change his ways and to start eating better and get more exercise. Our plant-based diet, rich in fruits and vegetables, is a perfect diet for protecting sexual health. We recommend that men who have high inflammatory factors avoid red meat and concentrate on eating fresh, wild fish, which is rich in anti-inflammatory omega-3 fatty acids, and that they take an omega-3 fatty acid supplement.

## Heavy Metal Toxicity

We live in a very toxic world in which people are exposed to all kinds of potentially damaging materials, from mercury in tuna to lead in consumer products imported from other countries to lead in the water from old pipes. High levels of heavy metals in the body can be quite toxic, but even moderate levels can cause inflammation, damage healthy cells, and cause a wide variety of symptoms indicating disrupted hormone production. We conduct a simple test called a urine challenge test to screen for heavy metals. If a man has high levels of lead or other toxic metal, we may recommend chelation therapy to remove it. Chelation therapy is a therapy that removes toxic metals from the body.

We evaluate the patient's medical history and laboratory test results before designing our treatment plan.

## WHEN TESTOSTERONE DECLINES

The average man experiences a 1.5% decline in testosterone every year past the age of 30. This may not sound like very much of a loss, but hormones are produced in such minuscule amounts that we measure them in nanograms (1 nanogram is equal to a billionth of a gram). Our cells are very sensitive to even tiny fluctuations in hormones, and over time, many men can feel the effects of lower testosterone levels. Some researchers in male health have likened the decline in testosterone in men to a "male menopause," or andropause. One school of thought, however, does not believe that the decline in testosterone in men is comparable to the mega-changes that occur in women during menopause.

Furthermore, some men lose testosterone at a faster rate than others. According to a 2007 study, weight gain is a major culprit. Adding just 4 to 5 points to your body mass index (BMI) produces a drop in testosterone levels similar to what naturally occurs over a decade. In other words, even a relatively small weight gain could age you in terms of your hormonal production. The same study found that men who developed chronic illnesses or took six or more medications had lower testosterone levels.

The study also confirmed what we see in our practice: healthy men have a slower and more gradual decline in testosterone than unhealthy men.

Regardless of their health, men today have lower levels of testosterone than those of previous generations. The Massachusetts Male Aging Study noted that a 60-year-old man in 2003 had 15% less testosterone than a 60-year-old in 1988. Furthermore, researchers noted that the decline "does not appear to be attributable to observed changes in explanatory factors, including health and lifestyle characteristics such as smoking and obesity."

So what is the cause of the decline? Outside influences that can cause a dip in testosterone include stress, but life really isn't that much more stressful today than it was a decade or so ago. There is, however, another more worrisome explanation—the impact of estrogenic chemicals in the environment on the male body. Some scientists suspect that lifetime exposure to xenoestrogens, estrogen-like compounds found in many commonly used chemicals including plastics, pesticides, and detergents, may alter normal hormone production. It's not outside the realm of possibility.

Many men today were weaned on plastic baby bottles, drink out of plastic water bottles or drink tap water polluted with chemical residues, play golf on pesticide-soaked greens, or eat food laden with pesticide residue. Furthermore, our food supply has been "hormone enriched" by food manufacturers more interested in their bottom line than in human health. Beef cattle are fed estrogen to fatten them up, and milk cows are given estrogen to promote milk production. (That's one reason why we recommend using only hormone-free meat products.) There's no hard evidence that xenoestrogens are responsible for the drop in testosterone in men, but scientists have also observed some hormonal aberrations in wildlife, specifically fish that swim in the waters we eventually drink.

When we suspect that a man is low in testosterone, we perform a hormone panel to check for free testosterone and SHBG. We then review his medical history to determine if he is a good candidate for testosterone replacement. We describe our approach to hormonal replacement in Chapter 9, "Hormone Makeover," and we educate him about the healthiest, most protective diet we know of (see Chapter 7, "Diet Makeover").

# SEX BUSTERS

### TOO MUCH STRESS

Men typically have two distinct reactions to stress. Some men are turned on by it, and these men generally find that sex is a great stress reliever. The "feel-good" endorphins pulsing through their bodies after they reach orgasm help to calm them down and soothe their nerves. Other men, however, find that feeling off kilter is very *un*sexy. They lose interest in sex when they are too stressed out. The problem is compounded in midlife men who may be experiencing occasional bouts of ED and are feeling stressed out about sex. Learning how to de-stress is a good first step to feeling sexy again. To learn how not to let stress get the better of you, see Chapter 11, "Mood Makeover."

## PERFORMANCE ANXIETY

Men who have problems with ED are often nervous that it will happen again long after the problem has been resolved. So they experience classic performance anxiety, which is almost a self-fulfilling prophecy. If you're worried about having erection difficulties, you will be so focused on your fears that you won't be able to concentrate on getting aroused and feeling sexy. Here again, communication with your partner is key to getting past your anxiety. We cover this in Chapter 6, "Sex Makeover."

## EXCESS ALCOHOL

Men who are stressed out may turn to alcohol as a way of coping. Although alcohol is reputed to "put you in the mood," in reality it's not great for your sex life. It raises the level of the hormone prolactin, which inhibits the production of LH, which turns on testosterone production. Heavy drinkers (generally defined as those consuming more than two alcoholic beverages daily) often have low levels of testosterone along with the resulting sexual problems.

## SMOKING

If you smoke, here's another great reason to quit. Studies show that men who smoke have lower sex drives, less frequent sex, and poorer sperm quality. Smoking is also a major risk factor for coronary artery disease, which leads to blockage of the small arteries that feed blood to the penis—a known cause of ED.

**LACK OF SLEEP**

Not getting enough shut-eye interferes with normal hormone cycling and can result in low testosterone. Furthermore, not sleeping makes you tired and stressed out, which is not conducive to good sex (see Chapter 5, "Not Getting Any Sleep . . . for All the Wrong Reasons").

**MEDICATION**

A surprising number of medications commonly prescribed to midlife men have sexual side effects, including lowering libido, making erections more difficult, and causing delayed ejaculation. Are you taking any medication that could be causing you problems? Review the list on page 31.

If you suspect that your medication is interfering with your ability to have sex, talk to your doctor. In some cases, switching to a different drug may make a difference.

## RELATIONSHIP PROBLEMS

At one time, the medical profession would dismiss cases of ED in relatively young men (between 40 and 60) as all in a guy's head, and in more mature men as just part of the annoyance of aging. Unaware of its physical causes, doctors frequently attributed ED to emotional problems, which was more often than not wrong. It left the man feeling bad himself, and his partner feeling that he could have sex if he just really wanted it badly enough. Now that we know the physiologic causes of ED, doctors often err in the other direction. They often ignore the fact that sometimes there is an emotional component stemming from the relationship. Anger, misunderstandings, and poor communication can turn a relationship toxic. In these situations, couples' counseling can be very helpful in terms of getting the relationship back on track.

## Concern About Partner

Both men and women in midlife undergo physical changes that can disrupt their sex lives. The vaginal atrophy, or thinning of the vaginal tissue, that occurs in many women after menopause can make intercourse painful. Some women experience a drop in libido. The men who care about them can see that their partners are not enjoying sex the way they used to and may even be experiencing discomfort. Fear and anxiety about hurting her may kick in, and a man may develop erection problems or not want to have sex at all. He may also interpret her difficulties as a rejection of him, causing him to withdraw.

We've also seen sexual problems develop when one or both partners have chronic illnesses, such as heart disease or arthritis. While there are people who are so ill that they can't have sex, many times finding a way to comfortably have sex can be helpful in that it makes people feel that they're back in the swing of things. The endorphins released during sex are also great natural painkillers. If you are worried about the impact of resuming sexual relations with a partner who has been ill, you both should talk to your partner's doctor.

---

### TUNE OUT, TURN ON

Do you watch three or more hours of television a day? Men who do are more likely to experience ED than those who watch an hour or less of television daily, according to a recent study published in the *American Journal of Medicine*. Researchers speculate that excess TV viewing means that you're not getting enough physical activity. The solution? Trade in your remote for a pair of walking shoes, and start doing some exercise.

---

## TOP SEX-BUSTING PRESCRIPTION DRUGS FOR MEN

### Antidepressants

Inhibit orgasm and decrease libido

**MAOI**

*moclobemide* (Manerix), *phenelzine* (Nardil)

**SEROTONIN INHIBITORS**

*fluoxetine* (Prozac), *paroxetine* (Paxil), *sertraline* (Zoloft), *escitalopram* (Lexapro), *venlafaxine* (Effexor)

**TRICYCLIC**

*amitriptyline* (Elavil), *nortriptyline* (Pamelor)

### Antihypertensives to Lower Blood Pressure

Can cause erectile dysfunction

**ACE INHIBITORS**

*benazepril* (Lotensin), *captopril* (Capoten), *enalapril* (Vasotec), *quinapril* (Accupril), *ramipril* (Altace)

**ALPHA-INHIBITORS**

*prazosin* (Minipress), *doxazosin* (Cardura)

**BETA-BLOCKERS**

*propranolol* (Inderal), *carvedilol* (Coreg), *metoprolol succinate* (Toprol XL), *atenolol* (Tenormin), *metoprolol* (Lopressor)

**CALCIUM CHANNEL BLOCKERS**

*diltiazem* (Cardizem), *nifedipine* (Procardia), *verapamil* (Calan), *felodipine* (Plendil)

## Diuretics

**THIAZIDES**

*chlorothiazide* (Diuril)

**ALDOSTERONE ANTAGONIST**

*spironolactone* (Aldactone)

## Cholesterol Lowering

Can cause erectile dysfunction

**STATINS**

*lovastatin* (Mevacor), *simvastatin* (Zocor), *atorvastatin* (Lipitor), *rosuvastatin* (Crestor)

**FIBRATES**

*gemfibrozil* (Lopid), *fenofibrate* (Tricor)

**H2 ANTAGONISTS**

*cimetidine* (Tagamet), *ranitidine* (Zantac)

## GI-Ulcer Drugs

Can cause erectile dysfunction

## Painkillers

**OPIOIDS**

*hydromorphone* (Dilaudid), *oxycodone* (Percodan), *fentanyl* (Fentora)

# PART TWO

# FRAZZLED, FAT, AND FATIGUED

## CHAPTER THREE

# WHEN YOU'RE FEELING DOWN

**HER**

*"I suffered from heart palpitations, dizziness, difficulty sleeping, and a whole lot of other unpleasant stuff. My doctor put me on antianxiety medication, which controlled my symptoms, but I felt dull and lethargic. I'm a business consultant—I've got a lot of high-powered clients, and I'd be sitting in meetings feeling really out of it. I wanted to get off the drugs."*

Barbara, an attractive, 52-year-old, married mother of two college-age children, sought our help to get off the medication she had been taking for anxiety.

Much of our practice revolves around helping people like Barbara better cope with mood-related problems, including anxiety and depression. Although they are considered to be different psychiatric disorders, both anxiety and depression have a common link—they can be caused or aggravated by chronic and intense stress.

Stress is not all bad. Some forms of stress can be stimulating if not exhilarating. Learning a new skill or mastering a physical challenge can force you to extend yourself beyond the norm, and that can be stressful. People run marathons, climb mountains, and tackle difficult tasks because they get some satisfaction out of the experience. But there's a real difference between good stress, which motivates you to achieve new heights, and debilitating stress, which weighs you down and can make you depressed and sick.

About one in eight Americans—more women than men—are diagnosed with clinical depression at some point in their lives. Anxiety affects about 4% of all Americans and can occur simultaneously with depression.

Some people are genetically predisposed to these problems, but others may succumb after a stressful period, such as the death of a loved one or a divorce. Mental health professionals used to make a real distinction between so-called event depression, which would often resolve on its own, and biological depression, caused by a biochemical imbalance. As we learn more and more about the biology of depression we now know that there is very little difference between the two: whatever the trigger, the end result is the same.

Mood problems are quite common, especially among midlife men and women. The physical changes of midlife, relationship issues, kids leaving home, work-related pressures, financial worries, health concerns, and the like can be extremely stressful.

Postmenopausal women are especially vulnerable to anxiety and depression, and sometimes it's difficult to figure out whether the symptoms are due to a true mood disorder or linked to hormonal imbalance. Whatever the root cause, mood problems can disrupt your life, hurt your health, and damage your relationships. Medication can help—up to a point. And we use it when we have to. But simply popping a few pills is not going to do the job, at least for most people. Very often, the real "cure" is a lifestyle overhaul—a Mood Makeover.

We gave Barbara a thorough physical examination to rule out any underlying health issues. We then interviewed her at length to learn about her habits and lifestyle. To her credit, she had built her successful consulting business from nothing but hard work. Although she loved her work and was used to the long hours, she had noticed that in recent years it was starting to take its toll. Like many people with stress-related symptoms, Barbara ate poorly and gravitated toward "sugar fixes" to maintain her energy, which only aggravated her stress symptoms. And like many people who feel overextended, Barbara wasn't happy about the extra pounds she had put on recently, but she felt she was too busy to deal with them. Now that her two daughters were away in college, she focused her energy on work, and she and her husband ate on the run. She didn't get enough exercise and rarely, if ever, truly felt relaxed.

## RX: A MORE HEALTHFUL LIFESTYLE

We developed a program to gradually wean Barbara off her medication and onto a more healthful lifestyle. First, we taught her the simple relaxation techniques we describe in Chapter 11, "Mood Makeover," such as deep breathing and stretching. Not only did she find these techniques to be surprisingly effective but she was delighted to report that she felt sharper and more mentally alert than she had in years. As we carefully weaned her off drugs we gave her a natural herbal remedy to promote better sleep. We have found that very often simply restoring normal sleep patterns can go a long way toward reducing anxiety and improving mood. We often try supplements first because they are milder than drugs, and they often do the trick. But if supplements don't work, we turn to prescription drugs (see page 82). We also put her on our standard Diet Makeover as well as a multivitamin and omega-3 fatty acid supplements. We don't recommend many supplements, but we do use a select group of supplements in our practice that we think are grounded in good science and are effective. In the case of mood problems, omega-3 fatty acids have been shown to be helpful. Barbara felt better fairly quickly.

### HIM

*"I thought that my wife was a nervous wreck, and I sought refuge in front of my computer. I worked all the time. I never realized that I was feeling just as bad as she was."*

As we got to know Barbara better we began to delve deeper into her life. We found out that although Barbara loved her husband, Tom, she was troubled by their relationship. Tom was a driven, successful entrepreneur who worked all hours of the day and night. Long after Barbara went to sleep, Tom would be up working at the computer in his den. Tom frequently suffered from migraine headaches and was irritable much of the time.

Barbara said that although on the surface they were fine, she felt a growing distance between her husband and herself. The couple rarely had sex, and when they did, Barbara felt it was purely mechanical and lacked any warmth or connection. As Barbara described it, she felt she was stuck in a "roommate marriage."

## DE-STRESSING YOUR MARRIAGE

To us, Barbara had described the textbook definition of the stressed-out marriage, or, as we also call it, the midlife marriage blahs. The marriage itself sinks into a bad mood. It's caused by a combination of factors—some physical, some emotional, and some circumstantial. In Barbara and Tom's case, once their kids went off to college, both partners tended to fixate on work. Their unhealthful lifestyle created physical problems that contributed to feelings of stress and tension in the relationship.

We thought that Barbara and Tom needed to approach this as a couple's problem. As it turned out, Tom was eager to get their relationship back on track, and he embraced our suggestions for improving his diet and getting enough sleep. And although his headaches didn't disappear, he began to see the connection between his lifestyle and his mood.

We had simple recommendations for specific ways that Barbara and Tom could de-stress their lives, improve their health, and revitalize their marriage, as we discuss in our Makeover chapters. And we discussed ways of nurturing intimacy outside the bedroom. For the first time in years, the couple actually sat down and had dinner together most nights, which was good for improving intimacy as well as their health. They also scheduled time to go out on dates and actually talk to each other. And they made it a point to spend time together at night before going to bed, as we recommend in Chapter 6, "Sex Makeover."

When a relationship begins to go south, it can be very stressful. Add to this the normal stressors we encounter daily, and many of us are walking around in a severely stressed-out state.

## THE BIOLOGY OF STRESS

Stress is not just a mental state; *it's a whole-body experience.* It can pervade all aspects of your health and well-being. And unless you learn to tame it, stress can leave you depleted physically and spiritually.

Your body's response to stress is controlled by the *autonomic* nervous system, but that's not all it does. The same system is in charge of many different organ systems in the body. It regulates your heartbeat, controls your breathing, and keeps your gastric juices flowing so you can digest your food. The best part is that it does all this without your having to think about it.

There are two main components of the autonomic nervous system: the *sympathetic* nervous system and the *parasympathetic* nervous system. Especially relevant, also, is the *enteric* nervous system.

The sympathetic nervous system (fight or flight) gets switched on when we're under stress. It's designed to protect us from danger, but as you'll see, it's a double-edged sword.

The parasympathetic system (rest and digest) is involved in healing, restoring, and repairing the body. It shuts down when we're in stress mode.

The enteric nervous system is a network of nerves centered in the digestive tract. It was recently discovered that these nerves produce some of the same chemicals found in the brain (so maybe there's something to "gut feelings" after all!), and it is in intimate communication with the sympathetic and parasympathetic systems—so much so that some regard it the third component of the *autonomic nervous system.* We mention it because of the profound effect that stress can have on the gut, from poor digestion to abdominal distress to poor absorption of nutrients.

When you're under stress, your body responds in a particular way. It prepares you for the worst. Your sympathetic system goes into high gear, switching the body into what is known as flight-or-fight mode. It's the same stress response system that became activated when our cavemen ancestors were being chased by predators. But in terms of typical modern-day stress—the demanding boss, the angry spouse, the unpaid tuition bill, the wait at the airport—more often than not it's overkill.

First, your brain orders a series of physiologic reactions that rev up the body. Your adrenal glands, located on top of the kidneys, are instructed to pump higher levels of stress hormones—adrenaline, noradrenaline, and cortisol—into your bloodstream. Your kidneys release renin, a hormone that raises your blood pressure. Your heart pumps faster, and blood is pulled away from your midsection and diverted to your legs to prepare for flight. Your blood sugar soars. Your pupils dilate so that you can see better at night. Your immune cells spew out pro-inflammatory chemicals to promote blood clots (to stop bleeding) and fight infection in case you are injured. You are geared up for action. You're supposed to be running for your life or fighting off a predator. And then, when you're out of danger, your parasympathetic system takes over, bringing it back down to normal.

Under ideal conditions, the production of stress hormones is shut down quickly, and your body can revert to handling its other business. And that means making new cells, repairing injured cells, and keeping your body systems humming along. But what if you don't get to burn off those stress hormones through activity, and you get stuck in stress mode? What if you are forced to sit and simmer at your desk, seething with anger? Or you spend the weekend sitting and seething in the airport lounge? And what if you find that you are frequently stressed out?

As you get older it becomes more difficult for your body to dispose of stress hormones. If you go into stress mode too often, over time, your cells become desensitized to the effect of stress hormones. Your adrenal glands don't get the proper feedback telling them to stop producing those hormones, and they keep pumping out more and more of them, even when you no longer need them. The net effect is that stress hormones stay in your system longer and longer, where they can do a great deal of mischief.

## Stress and Sex

In the brain, high levels of cortisol, in particular, are associated with imbalances in neurotransmitters, such as serotonin, acetylcholine, and dopamine—chemicals that allow brain cells to communicate with one another and to control mood and behavior. The wrong balance of these neurotransmitters—too much of one, or too little of the other—can lead to depression and anxiety. Antidepressants and anti-anxiety medication all target one or more neurotransmitters.

Stress can also affect your sex life, both directly and indirectly. When you are in stress mode, you're thinking about survival, not sex. This makes sense from an evolutionary point of view—when our cavemen ancestors were running away from predators, it wouldn't have been helpful for them to be distracted by thoughts of sex. Men require some input from the parasympathetic system to get and maintain an erection—it can't happen unless the blood vessels relax. If the parasympathetic nervous system is constantly overridden by the sympathetic nervous system, it's going to hamper a man's ability to have an erection. Furthermore, when you're in stress mode, your adrenal glands are so busy making stress hormones that they can't focus on their other jobs, which include making sex hormones. When the ovaries shut down after menopause—and, to a lesser extent, when the testes slow down during andropause—the adrenals help compensate for the loss by making estrogen and testosterone. Very stressed-out people don't have this reserve of sex hormones, and they are more likely to be hardest hit by menopause and andropause.

Without enough sex hormones, especially testosterone, you're not going to be thinking about sex. Not to mention the fact that when you're stressed out and feeling revved up all the time, it puts you in a very bad mood. And that has got to affect all aspects of life, especially your personal relationships.

It's not surprising that stress would have such a profound impact on mood—you know how lousy it can make you feel. What is remarkable, however, is the damage that unrelenting stress can inflict on every single organ system, from your brain to your heart to your bones to your immune system. Excess stress can make you age faster, and it can even make you fat.

41

## Stress and Obesity

When some people are under stress, they try to make themselves feel better by turning to "comfort food," which tends to be loaded with fat and sugar. As it turns out, this may be the worst thing they can do in terms of their weight and their health. Scientists have recently discovered a biochemical link between stress, weight gain, and prediabetes.

Researchers at Georgetown Medical Center tested the effects of chronic stress and weight gain in mice, especially around their midsection. Similarly to humans, when they are under stress, mice (and other animals) show marked changes in their body chemistry—changes that can make them fat. In one study, two groups of mice were subjected to ten minutes of stress every day: nothing terrible, but enough to make a mouse nervous. One group of stressed-out mice was fed a normal diet of mice chow. The other group was fed a high-fat high-sugar diet. Here's why this study is interesting: the mice eating the normal diet did not show an increase in abdominal fat. They remained trim and healthy.

The mice fed the high-fat high-sugar diet produced more belly fat, along with higher levels of a molecule called neuropeptide Y, which is known to stimulate the development of more fat cells, especially around the belly. Belly fat is one of several risk factors for prediabetes or metabolic syndrome, a condition characterized by a cluster of symptoms, including high blood pressure, elevated blood sugar, and insulin resistance. After three months, the mice on the high-fat high-sugar diet had indeed early signs of metabolic syndrome, which is also epidemic among American adults.

The takeaway message here is this: whether you're a mouse or a man (or a woman!), when you're under stress, your body produces chemicals that, when combined with a bad high-fat high-sugar diet, can make you hold on to fat, especially around your midriff. But, if you are careful not to succumb to eating bad food, you can avoid that stress-related weight gain.

In other words, the good news is that *diet can be protective against the negative effects of stress.*

## Stress and Your Aging Brain

Most of you have probably heard of antioxidants, vitamins, and phytochemicals (substances found in plant-based foods) that are reputed to keep us healthy and slow down the aging process. Antioxidants play a specific role in the body: they protect us against free radicals—substances that are naturally produced by the body and are a waste product of energy production. Free radicals need to be tightly controlled or they can cause a great deal of harm in the body. In particular, they promote inflammation, which can destroy healthy cells and tissues.

Free radicals target the mitochondria, the energy-producing structures of the cell that provide your body with fuel. As you age, the mitochondria die off, leaving cells with less energy to perform the same amount of work. Recently, some scientists have hypothesized that the loss of mitochondria is responsible for what we know as normal aging in the brain and everywhere else in the body.

The memory center of the brain, the hippocampus, is especially vulnerable to free radical damage and inflammation. Some scientists speculate that age-related memory loss—the "where did I put the keys?" phenomenon—is actually a result of a lifetime of stress-related inflammation. Stress can also raise levels of homocysteine, an amino acid produced by the body that if elevated can increase risk for Alzheimer's disease and stroke. Interestingly, elevated homocysteine can impair mental performance.

## Stress and Your Heart

Heart disease is still the Number One killer of men and women in the Western world, and here, too, stress can be a major culprit. As discussed earlier, stress hormones also promote free radicals and inflammation, which can also damage coronary arteries and lead to coronary artery disease.

Your mood can also have a profound effect on the health of your heart. Pent-up feelings of anger and hostility are associated with an increased risk of heart disease. There is also a strong link between depression and heart disease. People who suffer from mild to moderate depression are two to three times as likely to have coronary artery disease as those who do not, and those who suffer from severe depression are at five times the risk of coronary artery disease and also are at increased risk of cardiac death. This is not surprising, considering that stress is often a trigger for depression, or that depression itself can be very stressful.

For the sake of your heart, it makes sense to get stress under control.

### Stress and Your Immune System

Have you ever noticed that when you are under a great deal of stress at work, at school, or at home, you tend to be more vulnerable to colds and other illnesses? It's not your imagination—there's a scientific reason. Chronic exposure to emotional stress can dampen your immune responsiveness, reducing the effectiveness of specific disease-fighting cells. In fact, there's a discipline designed to study this phenomenon; it's called psychoneuroimmunology, and it is the foundation of mind-body therapy.

Studies show that a relationship marked by anger and hostility can weaken your immune system and make you more vulnerable to a variety of illnesses and possibly even cancer. Furthermore, older couples are more at risk of experiencing these negative changes in immune function, possibly because they are starting off with weaker immune systems. This is true not only of couples with marital problems; even relatively happy couples suffer a decline in immune function when they engage in heated arguments. In fact, one intriguing study showed that even a typical argument between a couple could delay the amount of time it took a wound to heal by at least twenty-four hours. This strengthens our case for the need for good communication in which both partners can talk openly to each other and resolve conflicts before they reach the shouting stage.

# A GOOD RELATIONSHIP: THE ANTIDOTE TO STRESS

Numerous studies have confirmed that a good marriage is protective against depression and heart disease, two problems closely linked to stress hormones out of control. And the flip side is also true: prolonged anger and hostility are toxic to your brain, your body, and your relationship.

Learning how to manage stress not only makes you feel good; it is absolutely essential for your health and well-being. And it is also of vital importance to your relationship.

A good relationship has proven health benefits; being married has been associated with better health and a longer life. The more you and your partner find common ground to support each other, the better for both of you. Cooking together and exercising together are healthful activities that also allow the two of you to be more connected. Most important, play together. The act of play and the experience of laughter have proven benefits to health and well-being.

CHAPTER FOUR

# THE LOWDOWN ON FAT

**HER**

*"The weight just crept up on me. I was a cheerleader in high school and a real fitness buff in my 20s, but the demands of work and caring for my family have made me neglectful of my diet. I don't watch what I eat, and I rarely get to the gym anymore. I used to care a lot about how I looked. I still do, but I don't think there's anything I can do about it. I think it really bothers my husband."*

**HIM**

*"Linda is very pretty, and okay, she may have put on a few pounds, but I'm still attracted to her, and I want to have sex with her, but we just seem to be growing further and further apart. She won't even get undressed in front of me anymore. I feel badly for her and for us."*

Jack came to see us for advice because he was upset about the state of his marriage to Linda, his high school sweetheart. Linda, now in her 40s, had put on quite a bit of weight recently, and she was clearly upset about it. Ideally, a husband should be able to say to his wife, "I still think you're pretty, I still love you, and I want to have a physical relationship with you," and that should do the trick. And vice versa. Men also put on their share of midlife pounds. But for many couples, weight has become such an emotionally charged issue; it's not that easy.

In these situations, couples' counseling can be very helpful. We talk to each spouse individually and then together. This gives the wife an opportunity to discuss how she feels about her weight. At the same time, it provides a platform for her husband to express how he's feeling, which is often quite different from his wife's assumptions.

After a few counseling sessions, Linda and Jack were able to express their warm feelings toward each other. This was a great relief to both of them, but it was only half the battle. On an intellectual level, Linda knew that Jack still desired her, but on an emotional level, she didn't feel very desirable. The other equally important task was to help Linda to feel comfortable again in her own skin—whether she was dressed or not. And that meant getting Linda to address the issue of her weight.

## HEALTHFUL WEIGHT, HEALTHFUL DIET

Weight is not only a cosmetic issue for women or men. It's a health issue—maybe *the* health issue— of our time. Being overweight increases the likelihood of developing heart disease, stroke, diabetes, high blood pressure, breathing problems such as asthma and sleep apnea, some cancers, osteoarthritis, and gallbladder disease. If you're obese, you face all the above risks plus a higher risk of dying at a relatively young age.

We talked to Linda about improving her diet for health reasons. But we also talked about how eating a more healthful diet would be good for Jack, too, even though he didn't need to lose weight. This presented another opportunity for the couple to work together.

We ended up prescribing our Diet Makeover to both Jack and Linda. It's a perfect meal plan to help you lose weight if you need to, but it's also a great way to get healthy and stay that way. In our conversations with Linda, we learned that she felt overwhelmed by the task of losing 20 pounds. We told Linda to stop following the scale. The real goal is a healthy diet; the decreased pounds will follow. Most of all, we stressed the connection between *eating well* and *feeling well*. Although Linda understood the importance of eating a good diet, there was a disconnect between that understanding and an awareness of how her poor eating habits were aggravating all the things that were bothering her.

We showed Linda how, despite her busy schedule, she could fit in at least one visit to the gym during the work week. We also encouraged Linda and Jack to begin the Exercise Makeover together on weekends because we have found that working out together is a great way for couples to reestablish intimacy.

Within a month, Linda had lost 8 pounds; more important, she began to feel more confident about how she looked. It took several more months for her to shed the 20 pounds she needed to lose to regain her health and her confidence. She never returned to the size 6 of her cheerleader days, but she looked trimmer and felt more attractive. Jack spent time assuring her that in his eyes she was still beautiful, and before long, he was happy to report that things were beginning to improve in the bedroom.

If Jack and Linda's story resonates with you, you're not alone. Both men and women tell us that gaining weight in midlife is one of their primary concerns—and yes, it often affects their sex lives.

## THE FAT EPIDEMIC

Some 60% of American adults are overweight, and about 25% are obese, which puts them at serious risk for many different diseases. In fact, the problems related to obesity make it the second leading preventable cause of death after smoking.

During midlife, the slowdown in metabolism makes it harder to maintain muscle and keep off excess fat. The (inevitable) undesirable weight gain can worsen hormonal problems. As we age we start to lose the muscle fibers that we need for strong, quick responses, such as jumping back from a car that runs a red light, or running from danger. Many of these are intertwined with nerve fibers, which die or recede with age, possibly leading to a loss of muscle tone.

When it comes to weight gain, stress is also a culprit. A stressed-out body can get stuck in overdrive. After a while, it's hard to shut it off on your own. The effect is an endless vicious circle, in which stress perpetuates a tense, anxious mood that often gets self-medicated with sweet, starchy foods and alcohol. This intensifies the metabolic changes from stress that cause fat to accumulate around the midsection and that can further deplete your body of sex hormones. To make matters worse, when your body is under constant stress, you lose interest in sex either because you are in a fight-or-flight mode or you're exhausted, feeling sluggish, and weighted down. And, of course, your self-image suffers, which is a real sex buster. Your mood dips, you make poor eating choices, and sex becomes a thing of the past.

What's worse, stress hormones have a catabolic effect, meaning that your body may break down more muscle than fat to burn as energy, and this causes increased storage of fat. As body fat increases, the percentage of muscle and bone to fat decreases, not only making it harder to keep weight off but also increasing the risk of many diseases, including osteoporosis. In both men and women, excess weight increases the risk of heart disease, diabetes, cancer, arthritis, and other so-called diseases of aging, which are often really a result of poor diet and a sedentary lifestyle.

## Her Weight Problems

Midlife (ages 40 to 60) is the most difficult time in a woman's life to maintain normal weight. In fact, some 65% of women between the ages of 45 and 54 are either overweight or obese. In addition, visceral fat—the most dangerous kind—is packed in a small region around your liver and other intra-abdominal organs. While the average woman may have 40 to 50 pounds of fat distributed throughout her body, somewhere between 5 and 10 pounds is intra-abdominal fat.

Women gain, on average, 5 pounds from perimenopause through menopause, and many put on much more. The majority of women see their weight creep up slowly, usually right around age 50. After menopause, a woman's weight tends to accumulate in the abdomen. We believe this is partly a function of the hormonal loss that characterizes menopause, when women's supplies of hormones—including estrogen, progesterone, and testosterone—are depleted. In particular, testosterone, which is present in both men and women, helps maintain muscle mass and bone mass. The loss of muscle mass results in decreased burning of fat mass and the increased percentage of body fat that is typical for postmenopausal women and midlife men. In addition, declining estrogen levels have been implicated as a contributory factor in the redistribution of body fat to the middle.

In women, excess body fat can lead to increased estrogen levels. At first glance this may appear like a good thing, but the evidence tells us that it isn't, particularly in regard to the risk of breast cancer. Some researchers theorize that the increase in breast cancer risk is due to an increase in estrogen feeding estrogen receptors on breast tumors. This may be so, but there are problems with that theory as a sole explanation. The science on this topic is still evolving, but our best determination is that the poor diet and lifestyle associated with obesity have a profound impact on the estrogen by converting it to the toxic metabolites linked to breast cancer and ovarian cancers. In addition, it has been our experience that these metabolites can have a detrimental effect on sex drive and also aggravate PMS and menopausal symptoms, although more research is needed to confirm these mechanisms.

We describe people who carry their weight around their middle as being shaped more like an apple than like a pear. Women whose excess fat tends to collect in the hips and buttocks are shaped more like pears, and while they may rage against their heavy thighs, they may be at lower risk for life-threatening diseases than their apple-shaped friends. Wider hips, on the other hand, may mean that you have bulkier bones and stronger thigh and buttocks muscles.

About 80% of women are more pear-shaped than apple-shaped before menopause. No matter what your body shape, the lower rates of heart disease that women under 50 enjoy in comparison with men disappear once menopause arrives. Talk about a change of life!

## His Weight Problems

For men, unfortunately, the equation is simple: the more weight a man gains from age 25 on, the shorter his expected life span.

In case that information wasn't enough to get you off the couch, we now know that a proven method to prolong the life span of living organisms—from fruit flies all the way to humans—is to eat a very low-calorie diet. Conversely, taking in more calories than you need, which results in being overweight and obesity over time, shortens the life span.

Fat cells interfere with the normal breakdown of hormones in the body. In men, excess fat can contain increased levels of the enzyme aromatase, which converts testosterone into estradiol. Estradiol can then be converted into a potent carcinogenic form of estrogen, which has been linked to prostate cancer. This aromatization process also lowers the levels of circulating testosterone, which has a negative effect on how a man looks and feels and makes him tired, flabbier, and feeling decidedly unsexy.

Testosterone is the hormone that is essential for sex drive and erectile function. The diseases that are brought on by excess weight, such as diabetes, high blood pressure, high cholesterol, and atherosclerosis, are exactly the same ones that can cause erectile dysfunction in men (see Chapter 2, "The Hard Truth About Sex for Him").

## WHY ABDOMINAL FAT IS SO DANGEROUS

While excess weight is unhealthy no matter where it is, carrying weight around your middle is the most harmful because deep abdominal fat is a biologically active organ. It secretes inflammatory chemicals that contribute to a buildup of hard plaque in the arteries, also known as atherosclerosis. Fat around the waist and abdomen is associated with a higher risk of high blood pressure, diabetes, early onset of heart disease, and certain types of cancers.

Weight within the abdomen dumps fatty acids into the bloodstream at a rapid rate. Fatty acids can affect insulin metabolism for better or for worse. The bad guys, trans fats (from hydrogenated oils) and saturated fats, turn on genes that desensitize your cells to insulin, which can lead to insulin resistance, which makes it increasingly difficult to control the amount of insulin released into the blood. Insulin resistance is a precursor to Type 2 diabetes. The good guys, healthful fats like omega-3 fatty acids, turn on genes that help promote insulin sensitivity. Simply picking the right fat can help send the right messages to your genes.

Here is another link between excess body fat and diabetes. Excess insulin can cause high blood pressure as well as unhealthfully high levels of cholesterol and triglycerides, some of the conditions that characterize metabolic syndrome, which often foreshadows diabetes and heart disease. The way to get the clearest picture of both your weight and your risk of heart disease and other inflammatory illness is to look at both your waist size (your waist circumference) and the relationship of your waist size to your hip size (your waist-to-hip ratio). For women, a waist circumference of more than 35 inches is considered in the high-risk category.

## How to Measure Your Waist-to-Hip Ratio

For both men and women, here's how to measure your waist circumference and waist-to-hip ratio. Take a measuring tape and wrap it around your waist at its narrowest point. Measure your hips with the tape measure at the widest point. Then simply divide your waist measurement by your hip measurement. A woman with a waist size of 33 and a hip size of 39.5 has a waist-to-hip ratio of 0.8. A man with a waist size of 39 and a hip size of 41 has a waist-to-hip ratio of 0.95.

Current guidelines say that women with waist-to-hip ratios of more than 0.8, and men with waist-to-hip ratios of more than 1.0, are at higher risk for diabetes

In fact, in a study that included more than 27,000 people in fifty-two countries, the waist-to-hip ratio was more strongly linked to heart attacks than the body mass index (BMI) in all eight ethnic groups that were studied.

Another recent study of nearly 6,800 men and women showed that a high BMI in midlife can mean a poorer quality of life with advancing age, including loss of strength and respiratory fitness. Not surprisingly, another study showed that being overweight and obesity in older men are associated with disabilities arising from cardiovascular issues. You can see examples of this as you see older people getting out of breath when they walk even small distances or attempt to climb stairs.

## Calculating Your Body Mass Index

In general, if you are 30 pounds or more over your ideal weight, you are considered obese. Calculating your BMI assesses your weight in relation to your height without regard to how much of your weight is muscle versus fat, which is an important distinction. To measure your BMI, you can either divide your weight in kilograms by your height in meters, squared, or you can multiply your weight in pounds by 705 and then divide that by your height in inches twice.

A BMI between 18.5 and 24.9 is considered best. If your BMI is between 25 and 29.9, you are considered to be overweight. A BMI over 30 is considered obese; and a BMI of 40 or above is considered morbidly obese, which raises the risk of death resulting from any cause by 50% to 150%.

Using the BMI, a man 5 feet 10 inches tall would be considered overweight if he is between 174 and 208 pounds, and obese at 209 pounds or more. A woman 5 feet 4 inches tall who weighs 140 pounds has a BMI of 24.1; if she weighs 160 pounds, her BMI is 27.5, which is considered overweight. And if that same woman's weight were 175 pounds, she would be considered obese according to the BMI.

Now for the good news. It turns out that the most dangerous fat is also the easiest to lose. In fact, when people lose about 10% of their body weight through controlling their dietary intake—especially by reducing their intake of animal fat—along with increasing their daily exercise, they often reduce their abdominal fat by as much as 30%. That's why keeping to the right weight is so essential at midlife—in addition to making you feel sexier, it also makes a tremendous difference to your cardiovascular and overall health.

## CHOLESTEROL: THE WHOLE STORY

We are the generation whose introduction to matters related to heart disease began with a discussion of cholesterol. At one time, doctors used to focus on the total amount of cholesterol in your body. We now know that that number tells only half the story. As you will see, the type of cholesterol you have is far more important than how much you have. It's time to go back to basics to understand exactly what cholesterol is and what it means to you in midlife.

Cholesterol is a soft, waxy substance that is found among fats circulating throughout your bloodstream and your cells. It is present in the cells of all animals. Your body makes cholesterol on its own; the rest comes from animal products like eggs, butter, cheese, meat, poultry (chicken, duck), fish, and milk with a fat content of 2% or more. Plant-based foods have no cholesterol in them. You have never heard anyone say, "I'm trying not to eat too many carrots because I'm watching my cholesterol," right?

Your body needs the right amount of cholesterol to produce cell membranes, some hormones, vitamin D, and the bile acids that help to digest fat. As you have heard through the years, unhealthful levels of cholesterol can lead to stroke or heart disease, specifically atherosclerosis, a condition in which fat and cholesterol are deposited on the artery walls in many parts of the body, including the coronary arteries feeding the heart. Like oil and water, cholesterol, which is fatty, and blood, which is watery, don't mix. The cholesterol made in the liver is combined with protein, making a lipoprotein, which carries the cholesterol through the bloodstream.

The two types of cholesterol are low-density lipoprotein (LDL), the bad kind, and high-density lipoprotein (HDL), the good kind.

If your LDL levels are too high—meaning there is too much circulating in your body—it can clog your arteries and increase your risk of heart attack and stroke. This bad cholesterol can slowly build up in the walls of the arteries in your heart and brain, forming plaque, which leads to atherosclerosis. If an artery already narrowed by plaque gets fully blocked, it can cause a heart attack or stroke. LDL is the cholesterol you are constantly trying to lower within your body. We recommend that you keep your LDL levels at 100 mg/dL or lower.

Not all LDL particles are equal. The so-called LDL activity is actually the sum of three groups of LDL: large, intermediate, and small. It is primarily the small particles that are considered to be the most damaging. We sometimes recommend that a patient get a special blood test that measures LDL size, not just total LDL, if we suspect a problem. HDL, the good cholesterol, carries cholesterol away from your arteries and takes it to your liver, where it's removed from your body. You can see why having high levels of HDL can help protect you from heart attacks. In fact, it appears that total HDL levels higher than 60 mg/dL may protect you against heart disease, whereas total HDL levels lower than 40 mg/dL for men and lower than 50 mg/dL for women may increase your risk for heart disease. We recommend that men aim for HDL levels of 50 mg/dL or higher, and that women aim for HDL levels of 55 mg/dL or higher.

Similarly to LDL, not all HDL particles are inherently protective. HDL is also the sum total of three groups of HDL: large, intermediate, and small. Conversely, in this case, only the largest HDL particles are helpful because they are the ones that scavenge and carry away the cholesterol. Once again, the only way to know whether you have beneficial HDL is to have a special blood test that measures HDL size.

## Triglycerides Count, Too

Triglycerides are a form of fat in the body, some of which is carried through the bloodstream and some of which is stored in fat tissue. Only a portion of your triglycerides are in the bloodstream. Merely having high blood triglyceride levels does not mean that you are on your way to atherosclerosis. But some lipoproteins that are rich in triglycerides also contain cholesterol, which causes atherosclerosis in some people with high triglycerides. Often people who have a high level of triglycerides may also have low levels of HDL, or may be at high risk for diabetes, both of which raise heart disease risk. So if your doctor tells you that your triglycerides are too high, you need to look more closely at your HDL levels, to make sure they're high enough, and at your LDL levels, to make sure they're low enough.

Triglyceride levels of 150 mg/dL or higher may increase your risk for heart disease. Many people with heart disease, diabetes, or both have high triglyceride levels. Once again, as with LDL and HDL, triglycerides are divided into three subgroups by size, with the large triglycerides being the most dangerous.

**The only accurate way to determine your cholesterol levels is to have blood drawn for a complete blood test. The test should specify your levels of HDL, LDL, triglycerides, and, if appropriate, subgroups as well. To accurately determine the level of triglycerides, you need to fast for 12 hours before having blood drawn—no food or liquids other than water.**

As for those quickie cholesterol testing places at health fairs and shopping malls, you can consider those as screening tests; so if you get results that indicate there is a problem, you need to follow up with comprehensive blood testing through your health care practitioner. That's the only way to get the full story.

## INFLAMMATION AND FAT

The biological process of inflammation is extremely complex. The immune system initiates an inflammatory process in response to injuries, as a way to slow down damage to the body. Think of how your skin itches and swells in response to a mosquito bite, or how your skin feels hot when it's sunburned. However, when inflammation becomes chronic, instead of limiting damage to the body, the ongoing inflammatory process causes the harm.

We now know that inflammation in the body is at the root of a great deal of disease, including cardiovascular and autoimmune disease. Asthma is also a result of inflammatory processes. Inflammation is at least as important as high cholesterol levels as a cause of heart disease.

In fact, in keeping with what we know about the dangers of fat around the waist, the most recent research has shown that this kind of fat is also associated with inflammation throughout the whole body, even when someone has a BMI and a waist circumference that are considered to be in the normal range. This tells us that abdominal fat, even in small quantities, can cause inflammation in the body.

Blood tests can determine levels of inflammation in the body. Elevated levels of high-sensitivity C-reactive protein (hs-CRP) indicate inflammation in the body; in fact, high levels of hs-CRP have been scientifically linked to a higher likelihood of heart attacks. Several researchers have linked high levels of hs-CRP to a higher likelihood of diabetes as well. The good news is that it is now possible to measure inflammation in the body and to determine whether or not you are insulin resistant and could be on your way to Type 2 diabetes. The even better news, as we've repeatedly said, is that the right lifestyle changes can prevent and even reverse many of these metabolic problems.

## IS DIABETES IN YOUR FUTURE?

Not surprisingly, health researchers describe the rate of diabetes in America as epidemic. Nearly 21 million children and adults in the United States have diabetes, which is about 7% of the population.

Diabetes is a disease in which the body either does not produce insulin at all or isn't able to use insulin properly. Insulin is a hormone that instructs the cells of the body to allow glucose (sugar) to enter them and give them energy—much as we put gas into the tanks of our cars to fuel them. Insulin is the hormone that helps convert sugar, carbohydrates, and other food into energy the body needs to function.

### TYPE 1 DIABETES:

This is the type in which the body is unable to produce insulin at all, so people with Type 1 diabetes must inject themselves with insulin. Only about 5% to 10% of Americans who are diagnosed with diabetes have Type 1 diabetes. This type used to be called juvenile diabetes because it was diagnosed in childhood. It is not a disease of lifestyle; rather, it is most commonly an autoimmune disease that destroys the pancreas.

## TYPE 2 DIABETES:

Type 2 diabetes is most often a disease of lifestyle. For people with Type 2 diabetes, their bodies are able to produce insulin but are unable to use it properly. They end up having both high insulin and elevated blood sugar levels. This is also referred to as insulin resistance. Type 2 diabetes is by far the most common form in the United States, accounting for up to 95% of all cases. It is generally treated with medication that lowers blood sugar, but sometimes it progresses to the point of needing insulin (hence, the insulin resistance we talk about is relative, and getting the body to respond with appropriate glucose levels requires more insulin than the body can make).

In addition to the nearly 21 million Americans with a form of diabetes, another 54 million of us have what is called prediabetes, or blood sugar levels (too high or too low) that forecast a very high likelihood of being diagnosed with diabetes within five to seven years. People with abnormally low blood sugar levels may also be considered to be prediabetic if their low blood sugar is generated by prolonged periods of elevated insulin levels because their bodies aren't responding to insulin properly and consequently increase insulin production.

However, for people who are prediabetic, research shows that with the right diet and exercise, it is possible to delay or even prevent Type 2 diabetes.

As for your blood sugar levels, the current recommendations are that your fasting level (after 8 to 10 hours) should be 100 mg/dL or lower as measured by a glucometer. If your fasting blood sugar is below 100 mg/dL, your chances of getting diabetes are low. A fasting blood sugar level over 100 puts you in the category of having a 10% to 15% chance of getting diabetes in the next seven years if you continue with the same diet and lifestyle.

In case you're not persuaded by what we have said so far about fat around the middle, researchers have found that this fat is also associated with the body's inability to process insulin and glucose properly. Abdominal fat is also associated with lowered levels of circulating testosterone in men.

## Diabetes, Your Heart, and Your Sex Life

On its own, diabetes is a serious disease. Moreover, it is closely linked to heart disease and stroke. In fact, about 65% of people who die of complications associated with diabetes die of either a stroke or heart disease. And think about this: adults with diabetes are two to four times more likely to die of heart disease than are adults who are not diabetic. For death resulting from stroke, the risk is about 2.8 times higher in adults with diabetes, and they're two to four times more likely to have a stroke than are adults who don't have diabetes.

In women with diabetes, deaths resulting from heart disease have increased 23% over the past thirty years, compared with a 27% decrease in women without diabetes. Deaths resulting from heart disease in men with diabetes have decreased by only 13%, compared with a 36% decrease in deaths resulting from heart disease in men who don't have diabetes.

As for men, one of the most common medical reasons for erectile dysfunction is diabetes: diabetic men are twice as likely to experience erectile dysfunction as are men without diabetes (see Chapter 2, "The Hard Truth About Sex for Him").

Women with Type 1 diabetes are twice as likely to experience sexual problems (such as impaired sensation and difficulty reaching orgasm) as are women without diabetes.

---

## KNOW YOUR NUMBERS

Normal blood pressure 120/80 mm Hg or lower

High blood pressure 140/90 mm Hg

Normal triglyceride level less than 150 mg/dL

High triglyceride level 200 mg/dL or higher

Normal blood glucose level (before eating) 70 to 100 mg/dL

Prediabetes blood glucose level (before eating) 100 to 125 mg/dL

---

### Diabetes and Ethnicity

It's true that people in certain ethnic groups, including African Americans, Latino/Hispanic Americans, Alaskan Natives, and Native Americans, have higher rates of diabetes than do Caucasians (white people). Why? Some people (called evolutionary biologists) who have studied these phenomena believe that a tendency toward diabetes developed among certain ethnic groups because of frequent episodes of starvation over time. Those individuals who adapted to lack of food by decreasing the amount of energy they used were able to survive, and they passed along this adaptation to the next generation. Unfortunately, the traits that helped these people survive without food seem to lead to insulin resistance when they have plenty to eat. That is, their metabolisms prepared them for doing without food for long stretches at a time. But our developed (some might say overdeveloped) world, with all its chips, dips, and fast food made up of sugars and starches, wreaks havoc with their metabolisms, driving the rate of diabetes in these populations sky high.

## WEIGHT: THE THIRD RAIL OF RELATIONSHIPS

### HER

*"My husband is more than 30 pounds overweight, and I'm really worried about him. No matter what I say, he won't go on a diet. And he gets very annoyed at me when I try to talk to him about his weight."*

We hear this complaint all the time from our patients. But the truth is, no matter how concerned you are about your husband's weight, it's *not* productive for you to lecture him about his need to go on a diet. He will respond by feeling both judged and controlled, which are two very negative emotions. This will make him resistant to even the most constructive advice.

The solution is for you to stop talking and to start acting. Try to engage your partner in a more healthful lifestyle that you do as a *couple*, as opposed to putting *him* on a diet. Tell him, "We're getting to a point in life where we should be healthier." And then start doing the things you need to do to make it happen.

### SHOP TOGETHER

Make food and a healthful lifestyle an important part of your relationship. Shopping for food should become a couple's event whenever possible. Make joint decisions about the food you bring into your house. Be willing to make compromises—especially at first—but do have a prepared list of what you need to purchase so that the shopping process is clear and efficient. You might be thinking, "My husband never wanted to grocery shop with me before; why will it be different now?" Sometimes it's helpful to start this process by making it fun in some way. For example, for the first few times, shop someplace unique, like trying out the farmer's market or a specialty store. Engage him in choosing some foods you don't typically prepare that he would like to try out. Also try combining the food shopping with something he likes to shop for, like "Let's check out that new farmer's market, and maybe we could also swing by the music store to pick up that new jazz CD you were talking about. In fact, we could listen to it over dinner tonight."

If your husband has a sweet tooth or enjoys snacks, you can steer him to more healthful versions of the foods he loves. Again, having him be part of the process and engaged in the choices will enhance the plan. Let him know that you don't plan to bombard him with sprouts and granola but that there are options other than eating the junk that might be hurting him. Remind him that this updated dietary approach is not about aesthetics; men often are not motivated by the concept of losing weight just to look better. Rather, the goal now is to improve things that are very tangible to having a better a quality of life: more energy, better clarity of thought, better sleep, better sex, and a lower risk of illnesses that are a big concern to baby-boomers and beyond.

Tell him that you hope the two of you can try some breakfast alternatives together, and ask if he is willing to join you in this health experiment. Select a lower-sugar, whole-grain, higher-fiber version of a cereal that he likes. If he tries to put a presweetened commercial trail mix into the cart, tell him that you would like to try an equally delicious but healthful trail mix that you can make on your own. (See the recipe for Dan's Trail Mix on page 145.) Or if he wants to buy soda, suggest that he mix a small amount of juice with sparkling water for a healthier drink. If he still insists on buying what he wants, leave it alone for the moment and just focus on adding the healthful food in the midst of the other stuff. You can't force your husband to make a positive change unless he wants to. In our experience, however, someone who begins eating in a better, more healthful way usually loses the sugar cravings that drive that person to eat those treats in the first place.

## COOK TOGETHER

Meal preparation can also become a couples event, which is good for your relationship and can even foster more intimacy. You may not be able to cook together every night, but even a few nights during the week or on weekends can be helpful in terms of keeping your husband involved in meal planning. If he has never been very active in the kitchen, keep it simple at first. Ask him to help you sharpen the knives and dice the onions. Remember that a little positive feedback goes a long way, so express appreciation of his involvement. The initial goal is to get him to dip his toe in the water so he can get a sense of the direction he might want to swim in. Keep it consistent until the joint preparations become second nature. Some couples find that having small dinner parties for friends really mobilizes their cooking team into action and prompts them to find an array of recipes that work for them.

## EXERCISE TOGETHER

Work on ways you both can get more physical activity, alone or preferably as a couple. Take walks together and go to the gym together. Buy your husband some sessions with a physical trainer at the gym to show him how to work out effectively. Or find a trainer who will work with both of you.

In addition to the workout routine we suggest for both of you, the best kind of exercise employs play of some kind, ideally with each other. This is the time to start couples tennis, ballroom dancing, cross-country skiing, golf, or whatever activity you thought you wanted to try back in the days when raising a family made it impossible to carve out that niche of time. Having an athletic activity you like to do together will also motivate the two of you to have a regular workout routine, because you'll find that the better shape you're in, the better you'll be at the activity.

The point is, this approach is for BOTH of you and for the good of your relationship, not just for the overweight spouse.

## CHAPTER FIVE

# NOT GETTING ANY SLEEP . . . FOR ALL THE WRONG REASONS

**HIM**

*"She was driving me crazy all night. First she's too cold, then she's too warm, then she's cold again. I kept turning the thermostat up and down. Neither one of us sleeps very well these days."*

**HER**

*"His snoring is so loud that I can't sleep. The whole bed vibrates from the noise! Most nights he sleeps in the den, and I hate it. I get lonely."*

If you're having difficulty sleeping (and we do mean *sleeping*) with your partner, you're not alone. Sleep problems are a very common complaint among our midlife patients. The problem can be so bad that many couples end up sleeping in separate rooms. A survey conducted by the National Sleep Association revealed that 23% of married couples sleep apart.

This is unfortunate. Beds are not just for sleeping. They're for cuddling, for late night or early morning talks, and, of course, for sex and intimacy. So if you're not spending time in bed with your partner, your relationship is likely to suffer. Our goal is to solve a couple's sleep problems so that we can keep the couple in the same room and preferably in the same bed.

The problem is not just snoring that keeps couples awake at night. Hormonal changes typical of midlife can drastically alter sleep patterns for both men and women. If one partner suffers from insomnia, or wakes up too early, or is restless, or too hot, or too cold, or is a very light sleeper, the other partner is likely to be losing sleep by default.

Even people who have no problem sleeping stay up until the wee hours of the night because so many distractions keep them from going to bed. As a result, today we get about 20% less sleep than our ancestors got a hundred years ago. In the candlelit world of our great-grandparents, there wasn't a whole lot to do after dark. People retired early, and they were healthier for it in terms of being less likely to develop the two modern killers of this century: heart disease and cancer. Of course, the life expectancy was shorter, but that was due primarily to poorer hygiene, infectious diseases, and the lack of antibiotics. Today, we live in a 24/7 world that never shuts down. Thanks to electric lights, all-night TV, the internet, and twenty-four-hour restaurants, we no longer associate night with sleep. Many of us drag ourselves into bed only when we are so tired that we can't keep our heads up any longer.

The result is that most of us are not getting the restorative sleep we need to get through the day and maintain our health. According to a 2002 report by the National Sleep Foundation, as many as 47 million Americans are walking around sleep deprived. The researchers found that many "problems and frustrations" that have become associated with American life, including road rage, stress, and obesity, may be linked to too little sleep. Indeed, the researchers believe that those of us who don't get enough sleep are more likely to be quarrelsome and to overeat than those of us who are well rested. Chronic lack of sleep is not conducive to a good relationship.

We now recognize that sleep deprivation exacts a steep toll on our physical and emotional health. It is often a contributing factor of the Big Three midlife problems: sexual dysfunction, weight gain, and mood problems. These problems are so closely related to sleep that it's often difficult to tell where one ends and the other begins. For example, insomnia is often a sign of depression, which can reduce sex drive. But insomnia can be due to any number of problems, including chronic pain, stress, or midlife hormonal changes. And all the above can leave you depressed. Furthermore, if you don't get enough sleep, you're at higher risk of developing several physical problems, including high blood pressure, heart disease, and obesity.

True, sleep is a time of winding down for the body, but when you're sleeping, your brain is surprisingly active. There are two different types of sleep. The first is known as NREM sleep. "NREM" stands for non-rapid eye movement activity. This is the most restful form of sleep. The other type of sleep is known as REM sleep. "REM" stands for rapid eye movement activity. Each type of sleep is important in its own way and serves different purposes. We typically have four to six sleep cycles per night where we move from NREM sleep to REM sleep. Each cycle consists of sixty to a hundred minutes of NREM sleep followed by a brief period of REM sleep.

Getting enough REM sleep is particularly important for learning, memory, and mood. Studies have shown that a lack of REM sleep can make us irritable and anxious and cause us to have difficulty concentrating. Interestingly, it can also cause us to overeat or lose our appetites. Clearly, there's something therapeutic about dreaming.

## UP ALL NIGHT? YOU'RE NOT ALONE

Sleep disturbances are very common among midlife people, for many reasons. Medications taken for chronic medical conditions, such as antihistamines for asthma or NSAIDs for arthritis, can disrupt sleep patterns. Many physical and emotional problems can cause sleep disturbances. So can taking antidepressants.

The hormonal changes that occur in men and women during midlife can also affect sleep patterns. We tend to think of hormones solely in terms of their role in the reproductive system, but in fact, hormones are critical for regulating normal sleep-wake cycles. Poor sleep is one of the first symptoms of perimenopause partially because of a drop in progesterone, a hormone that promotes feelings of well-being. Low levels of progesterone can contribute to stress and anxiety, which are not conducive to a good night's sleep.

Moreover, hormones govern our internal biological clock, which tells our bodies when to sleep and when to wake up. There's a reason why we turn out the lights when we go to sleep. Darkness triggers the production of melatonin by the pineal gland, a pea-sized structure embedded deep within the brain. The release of melatonin lowers our body temperature, slows our heart rate, and makes us sleepy. Daylight inhibits the production of melatonin, which is why we tend to awaken around dawn. Electric lights can also suppress melatonin production, which is another reason why the 24/7 nonstop lifestyle can cause sleeping disorders.

Levels of melatonin are highest during childhood. They drop off during adolescence, triggering hormonal changes and puberty. Melatonin production slowly declines as we age, but there is a steep drop at around age 50. You won't be surprised to know that age 50 is also the time when people begin to experience sleep disturbances. Some people have found that taking melatonin supplements can restore normal sleep patterns, and we'll discuss how to use melatonin, other over-the-counter supplements, and prescription medications later in this chapter.

Most sleep problems can be solved by lifestyle changes, diet, or redecorating. No, it's not a typo, we did mean to say "redecorating." The right bed and the right surroundings are critical for a good night's sleep, but we'll get to that later.

In order to fully appreciate the importance of sleep, you need to understand the good things it does for your body.

## SLEEP CAN BE REJUVENATING

There are many theories about the purpose of sleep—including why we need it and what it does. Nevertheless, until recently, the importance of sleep was minimized. Biologists went as far as to suggest that the only purpose of sleep was to force our prehistoric ancestors to lie low at night so they were protected from predators. We now know that there is much more to sleep than was once believed.

Sleep gives your body time to repair and renew itself. Your body systems wind down during sleep. Your metabolism slows. Your heart rate drops, and so does your blood pressure. Your level of human growth hormone rises during sleep, and this stimulates the repair of old cells and the production of new ones. (Interestingly, exercise is another way to boost human growth hormone.) So, in a sense, sleep is a period during which your body de-ages itself. Missed sleep is a missed opportunity for rejuvenation.

Sleep is also a way of dealing with the stress of the day. Your brain is surprisingly active during sleep, and there is some evidence that while you sleep you are actually sorting through the events of the day, processing information and even solving problems. During sleep, levels of neurotransmitters—important chemicals that help you think and learn and that regulate mood—are normalized. In contrast, when you don't get enough sleep, your body pumps out higher levels of cortisol, a hormone normally released during times of stress. This could explain why people who miss sleep are often so irritable and moody! And you know from Chapter 3, "When You're Feeling Down," the damaging effects that stress hormones can have on all the systems of the body.

The sleep-weight connection is particularly intriguing. Studies show that people who routinely don't get enough sleep, which means about seven hours a night, are at greater risk for obesity. The question is why? Recently, scientists have discovered that sleep deprivation alters the production of metabolic hormones that regulate appetite, resulting in feelings of hunger. It's hard to refrain from eating if you're constantly hungry, especially if you are also fatigued from not sleeping. That's why we tend to overeat when we're tired.

Furthermore, chronic lack of sleep may increase the risk of adult-onset diabetes, which is also associated with obesity. According to a 1999 study published in *The Lancet*, during a period of sleep deprivation, men's blood sugar levels took 40% longer to drop after they had eaten a high-carbohydrate meal, and they were less able to respond to insulin, the hormone that regulates blood sugar and fat metabolism. Sleep deprivation also resulted in cortisol levels that were higher than normal and thyroid-stimulating hormone levels that were lower than normal. Notably, the hormone levels of sleep-deprived people are similar to the hormone levels of much older people. Sleep is rejuvenating. Sleep deprivation appears to have precisely the opposite effect.

If you're losing sleep because you or your partner is having problems getting to sleep or staying asleep, it's important for both of you that you deal with it. Rest assured, there are things you can do to ensure that both of you get the good night's sleep you need. The first step to solving the problem is getting to its root cause. There are numerous medical and emotional factors that could be keeping you up at night.

## WHAT'S KEEPING YOU UP?

Everyone experiences an occasional bout of insomnia or difficulty falling or staying asleep. According to a recent study, as many as 100 million Americans have suffered from insomnia at some point in their lives. Both men and women are affected by insomnia, although women seem to be slightly more susceptible to the problem. Transient insomnia lasts for only a few nights and is usually caused by a specific trigger, such as jet lag, excitement, illness, temporary stress, or a change in sleep schedule. It usually resolves on its own.

Short-term insomnia lasts up to three weeks and is often due to more prolonged stress or worries, the death of a loved one, a job change, or a divorce. If not addressed, short-term insomnia may develop into a chronic problem.

Insomnia is considered to be chronic—and should be taken seriously—if it persists for more than a month. It could be a symptom of an underlying medical condition, including depression. Many women are awakened night after night by hot flashes, which can leave them exhausted the next day. For these women, a medical intervention such as hormone replacement therapy can be a true lifesaver.

Restless legs syndrome (RLS) is another common cause of insomnia that strikes during midlife. RLS is characterized by an uncomfortable urge to move your legs, and it gets worse when you are lying down. People with RLS may experience a tingling feeling—and in some cases pain—in their legs. If RLS kicks in when you're trying to fall asleep or during sleep, it can disrupt your sleep. The cause of RLS is unknown, although it is often associated with other medical problems, such as peripheral neuropathy, diabetes mellitus, anemia, or rheumatoid arthritis. Mild exercise can relieve RLS symptoms, but strenuous exercise can actually worsen the condition. So don't overdo your workout. Prescription medications may also help. If RLS is keeping you awake, you should see your doctor.

Teeth grinding—bruxism—is another common problem that can keep you up at night, not to mention what it does to your teeth and gums. In severe cases, bruxism can cause headaches and problems with your neck and jaw. Treatments include dental appliances that hold your mouth in place and stop the grinding. Bruxism is usually associated with stress, although it could also be due to poorly aligned teeth. If you suffer from bruxism, make an appointment with your dentist to determine the root cause. If you suspect that stress is your problem, turn to Chapter 11, "Mood Makeover." Your dentist will be able to treat the problem; the Mood Makeover will help eliminate the stress that is causing it.

Not sleeping is hazardous to your health. If you have chronic insomnia, you should see your doctor for an evaluation, because today, fortunately, there are some excellent treatments for insomnia. These treatments include some state-of-the-art nonaddictive sleep medications that work well without making you groggy. We prescribe these sleep aids from time to time because, in some cases, just getting back on track is all that's necessary to restore normal sleep patterns.

## SNORING: THE COUPLE'S NIGHTMARE

Get a group of midlife couples together and ask them how many of them are still sleeping in the same room. You'd be surprised by how many are spending at least some of the night apart these days. Why? One partner is being kept up by the other partner's snoring. More often than not, it's a woman complaining about a man.

Snoring is probably the most common of all sleep problems, affecting about 40% of all midlife people. We tend to think of snoring as a male problem, but in fact, women are starting to catch up. About four out of ten men snore, compared with three out of ten women. Snoring often leads to separate bedrooms and a loss of physical and emotional intimacy. This can put a real strain on a relationship.

The medical definition of snoring is noisy breathing through the mouth or nose during sleep. Every one of us snores on occasion, particularly if we are suffering from a cold or seasonal allergies. I'm sure that most of you have at one time or another elbowed your partner in the middle of the night to get him or her to quiet down. In the case of mild snoring, usually just turning over will stop it, or at least quiet it down. Snoring is considered a more serious problem if it doesn't stop when the person shifts sleeping position. Severe snoring is often the result of a condition called sleep apnea, in which breathing—and sleep—are actually interrupted, sometimes hundreds of times a night. Sleep apnea requires medical attention (see page 77).

In many cases, snoring, in and of itself, is not a problem for the snorer, unless it is so loud and persistent that it keeps waking the snorer up. More often than not, it's the bed partner who is suffering.

## What Is Snoring?

Why is it possible for someone to breathe perfectly normally (and quietly) during the day but snore loudly at night? The explanation is that sleep is a time when the muscles of the body become relaxed, and that's what causes the problem. During deep sleep, the muscles in the throat relax, and the airway, which brings oxygen to and from the lungs narrows. Snoring is the fluttering sound created by the vibrations of tissues against each other in the back of the throat and nose. The tissues involved in obstructing the airway and vibrating against each other can be the throat itself, or the tonsils, the adenoids, the soft palate (the roof part of the mouth), or the uvula (the little piece of flesh that hangs down from the soft palate). What causes the airway to narrow to the point at which it causes you to snore? Many factors contribute to snoring, some of which are induced by lifestyle. The severity of snoring depends on several factors, including the degree of obstruction, the anatomy of the throat, and even what the snorer ate or drank that night.

The good news is that there are lots of ways to treat snoring. Some people may require medical treatment, but many of the most effective methods are simple things you can do on your own. The first step is to figure out what's causing your snoring problem.

Structural abnormalities, such as a deviated septum or nasal polyps, either of which can block your nasal passage, can cause snoring. So can larger-than-normal adenoids or tonsils or a long uvula or a soft palate, which can obstruct the airways in your throat and cause vibration during breathing. (Many bed partners of snorers complain that the vibration from snoring is far more annoying than the noise.) If you suspect that you may have a problem with your nose or throat, you should be evaluated by an otolaryngologist—an ear, nose, and throat specialist—who will check for any structural problems. Men tend to have narrower air passages than women, which is why men are more prone to snoring. As you age, your throat becomes narrower and the muscle tone in your throat decreases. Any condition that can cause a blockage in your nasal airways, such as allergies, asthma, colds, or sinus infections, can induce snoring. Ironically, the antihistamines you may be taking to alleviate the congestion can actually cause snoring by relaxing the throat and tongue muscles.

## Ten Simple Ways to Say Goodnight to Snoring

Sometimes making simple changes in your routine or lifestyle can quickly solve your snoring problem. If your snoring is not severe, we recommend trying these simple steps first before seeking medical help.

## LOSE WEIGHT

Excess weight and fatty tissue in the neck can cause your throat to narrow. If you are overweight, especially if you have a double (or triple) chin, losing weight can help reduce or even eliminate snoring. People are very surprised by how the loss of just a few pounds can make a real difference in their breathing and snoring. If you lose 10 pounds, you will shrink your neck size by 1 inch, and that may help get your snoring under control.

## SKIP THE NIGHTCAP

Alcohol relaxes throat muscles. If you tend to drink before bedtime, don't. You'll sleep more soundly but make less noise.

## DON'T SMOKE

Smoking or exposure to secondhand smoke relaxes the throat muscles and also causes congestion in the nasal passages and lungs. If you smoke, you need to stop for a lot of reasons, including the fact that it causes snoring.

## AVOID ANTIHISTAMINES

If a stuffy nose is keeping you up, there are alternatives to antihistamines. We often recommend an old-fashioned remedy that works extremely well: inhaling hot steam with eucalyptus. It's as easy as boiling water. Really! Just fill a pot with water and bring it to a boil. Throw in some eucalyptus oil or fresh eucalyptus leaves, and let it sit for a minute or two. Carefully remove the pot from the stove, place it on a table, and inhale the vapor for about five minutes. You can put a towel over your head and the pot to make a tent. Just be careful not to burn yourself. Many people find that steam clears their nasal passages without drying them out, allowing them to fall asleep and stay asleep.

## SLEEP ON YOUR SIDE

If you tend to snore when you sleep on your back, try sleeping on your side. If you can't seem to break the habit of sleeping on your back, try the old tennis ball trick.

Sew a sock to the back of your pajama top. Put a tennis ball in the sock. Then go to sleep. If you attempt to lie on your back, you will be awakened by the pressure of the tennis ball. In time, you will naturally begin to sleep on your side, and the tennis ball will no longer be needed.

### AVOID SLEEPING PILLS

We prescribe sleeping pills for some patients—but with caution if they snore, because these drugs relax throat muscles and may increase snoring.

### SLEEP ON A FIRM PILLOW

Sleeping with a very soft pillow that doesn't support your head can increase the angle of your neck, which in turn can force your tongue and jaw to fall backward in your throat. This will block your airway, causing you to snore. You may have seen advertisements for "antisnoring" pillows that are purported to be specifically designed to reduce snoring. These include memory foam pillows, and even pillows filled with buckwheat. We've had mixed reviews from patients as to whether these pillows work any better than a standard firm pillow. Some patients have reported good results from one or more of these pillows, but some have found them to be very uncomfortable. Our best advice is to try out a few pillows for yourself and see if any of them work for you.

### ELEVATE YOUR BED

Elevate the head of your bed by about four inches. This position may make breathing easier and pushes your tongue and jaw forward. You can buy a foam wedge to put under the mattress, or you can place rolled-up towels underneath the mattress so that the head of the bed is elevated. It's better to elevate the entire head of the bed than to use several pillows to achieve the same elevation, because pillows can crimp the neck and actually contribute to snoring.

You can also invest in an adjustable bed that allows you to set the head of the bed to the correct angle. Most of these beds have dual controls so that your partner can set the other side of the bed to whatever works best for him or her.

## AVOID HEAVY MEALS AT NIGHT

Late-night eating also promotes snoring because the process of digestion also re-laxes the throat and tongue muscles. If you must eat, avoid high-fat dairy products—such as ice cream—before sleeping. Milk products can keep mucus from draining properly—yet another reason not to eat ice cream at night.

## AVOID SPICY FOOD AT NIGHT

Spicy food can trigger indigestion, which could lead to snoring.

## GET SOME EXERCISE

Poor overall muscle tone and lax muscles contribute to snoring problems. Exer-cise will tone you—and the tissues that are involved in snoring—up. But don't exercise too late in the evening; it could keep you up. Try to do your workout at least three hours before bedtime. (See Chapter 8, "Exercise Makeover.")

## LEARN TO PLAY A WIND INSTRUMENT

Believe it or not, playing a wind instrument can help improve the muscle tone of the roof of your mouth and strengthen your upper airways. Studies have shown that playing one wind instrument in particular, the Australian didgeridoo, can be particularly helpful for people who snore or who have respiratory problems. We're not kidding. It really works. (Although other wind instruments have not been studied, there is no reason to believe that they won't work as well.)

## EXPLORE OVER-THE-COUNTER OPTIONS

Various over-the-counter products are helpful in reducing snoring. These include nose sprays that moisten your nasal passages, antisnoring throat sprays that lubri-cate and tone your throat muscles, chin strips that reposition your tongue and jaw to open your airways, and special pillows that force you to sleep on your side. They don't work for everyone, but they work for enough people that we feel that they are worth a try.

## Get Help

If these simple things don't give you (or your partner) relief, you need to consult your physician, who will check for structural problems. If you have an anatomical problem that is causing your airways to narrow, such as a larger-than-normal uvula, or excess throat tissue, you may want to consult a dentist who specializes in making dental appliances designed to reduce snoring. Several oral devices can be worn at night that open up the airway by repositioning the tongue and jaw. Some are worn inside the mouth, like an orthodontic appliance, and some are fitted around the head and chin to adjust the position of the lower jaw. These devices can be extremely effective in opening up the airway and reducing snoring.

Depending on your problem, you may also need to see a sleep specialist, who may suggest that you spend a night at a sleep clinic where your sleep patterns can be observed.

In some cases, your doctor may recommend throat or nose surgery to correct the problem. These procedures can be painful, and they are not always successful.

For example, in snoreplasty, the physician injects a scarring agent into soft tissue to stiffen the palate and thereby improve airflow. In a 2003 study of patients undergoing this procedure, most patients experienced some reduction in snoring after nineteen months, although 18% reported they had relapsed.

Somnoplasty is a procedure in which radiofrequency signals are used to heat a thin needle, which is inserted into excess throat tissue to open up the airway. A 2000 study conducted at the Birmingham Heartland's Hospital in the United Kingdom found that the success of this procedure is directly related to body mass index (BMI)—that is, the leaner you are, the better the result. According to this study, somnoplasty is not an effective treatment for severely overweight people with a BMI of 30 or more (see page 53 for information on the BMI).

Uvulopalatopharyngoplasty (UPPP), the most aggressive treatment, is the surgical removal, by laser or scalpel, of excess throat tissue. The surgeon may also remove tonsils or adenoids if they are narrowing the airway and may even reconstruct your jaw if necessary.

This is not a trivial procedure and should not be undertaken lightly. In a 2005 Swiss study of 146 patients who had a modified UPPP between January 1992 and December 2003, about three-quarters of the patients showed improvement in their snoring, and 85% were pleased with the result. Nevertheless, 23% had some long-term complications, including chronic dry mouth or difficulty swallowing. And 27% of the patients said that if they had to do it over again, they would not have the procedure. Our take is that this is a procedure of last resort, to be used only if nothing else works.

## SLEEP APNEA

If you have a severe snoring problem, it is critical that you get a thorough examination to determine if you have sleep apnea. The word "apnea" is derived from the Greek word for "want of breath," which aptly describes this potentially life-threatening condition. About 4% of men and 2% of women have sleep apnea. If you have sleep apnea, your breathing is briefly interrupted as often as hundreds of times each night. Sleep apnea is characterized by a distinctive pattern: snoring followed by a short period of silence that ends with a loud gasp as you start to breathe again. The sound of your bed partner gasping for breath can be extremely distressing. Very often, spouses are the ones to first diagnose the problem and urge their loved ones to get treatment.

If you suspect you have sleep apnea, you need to see your doctor for an evaluation. The frequent interruptions in sleep prevent the apnea sufferer from getting enough rest. Not surprisingly, people with apnea typically experience daytime sleepiness and often are irritable, suffer from morning headaches, and have diminished sex drive. Furthermore, sleep apnea significantly increases the risk of heart attack and stroke.

The most common type of sleep apnea, obstructive sleep apnea, occurs when the tongue or other soft tissue blocks the airway, narrowing it to the point at which it compromises breathing. The brain is deprived, albeit briefly, of oxygen, and carbon dioxide builds up in the blood, which sends a message to the brain that you need to breathe again. This causes the brief awakenings and the gasps for air.

If your doctor suspects that you have sleep apnea, he or she will send you to a sleep laboratory for a special test called a polysomnography. The test is usually conducted at night and monitors your sleep patterns as well as physiologic responses, such as heart rate, breathing, and blood pressure. Once the diagnosis of sleep apnea is made, your doctor will suggest treatment options. The risk factors for sleep apnea are similar to those for snoring. There is often a hereditary component, but obesity also plays a major role. In the case of mild apnea, weight loss often helps, as do our other conventional suggestions for dealing with snoring, such as sleeping on an elevated mattress, using a firm pillow, and employing dental appliances to open up the airway. Surgery is also an option, but once again, the results are unpredictable.

Many apnea sufferers find relief by using a nighttime breathing device called a nasal CPAP. The abbreviation stands for continuous positive airway pressure. A CPAP mask that is attached to a pump is placed over the mouth and nose of the apnea sufferer. Air pressure is continuously pumped through the mask to open the airway. Although the nasal CPAP works well for many people, it can take some getting used to. Not everyone can tolerate it, and some bed partners don't like the "white noise" emitted by the machine.

## THE RIGHT MOOD FOR SLEEP

In order to get the restorative sleep you need to look and feel good, you must live a lifestyle that is conducive to sleep. The first and most important step is for you and your partner to decide to make sleep a priority in your lives. To do this, you must establish a sleep routine. Try to get to sleep at the same time every night and wake up at the same time in the morning. Don't do things that will sabotage your sleep. Avoid drinking caffeinated beverages, such as coffee, tea, and cola, after two o'clock in the afternoon. If you have to smoke, don't smoke at night.

Nicotine is a stimulant. Try not to eat a heavy meal at night, and avoid spicy foods and foods high in sugar. If you are hungry, have a light snack before bedtime: a piece of fruit, a small salad, a protein shake, or a home-baked oatmeal cookie.

The bedroom is a couple's sanctuary. Your bedroom should be a place where you and your partner can enjoy spending time together. Your bedroom should be neat and serene. It should not be a place where you pay bills, store files, or stash the fax machine. Make your bed every day, even if you don't get around to doing it until just before bedtime. That way, the bed will feel neat and inviting—not a reminder of the things you didn't get around to doing that day. Fresh flowers or scented candles (especially lavender-scented ones) will help make your bedroom an oasis. If you've ever stayed in a room at a good hotel or resort that you particularly liked, think about the elements that made the room special, and try to incorporate them in your bedroom at home.

If you live on a noisy street or have noisy neighbors, try using a white noise machine to mask annoying sounds. Many people find white noise to be very soothing.

Light alters the way your brain produces the hormones that regulate your sleep-wake cycles. Keep your room as dark as possible. If outside light is a problem, use heavy curtains or drapes. Keep TVs and computers OUT of the bedroom, because the light from the screens can disrupt melatonin production, and that will keep you awake.

Music, on the other hand, is okay. In fact, listening to soft music is a wonderful way to wind down. Keep a stack of your favorite CDs in your bedroom, or program your MP3 player with special selections for nighttime listening, but make sure it is programmed to switch off automatically.

The bed must be comfortable for both partners. Fortunately, there are many beds on the market today that accommodate the different needs of partners. Some have dual controls that allow you to adjust the firmness of the mattress as well as the angle of the head or end of the bed. If one partner is a restless sleeper, consider getting a special mattress that absorbs pressure, so you don't feel it move every time your partner adjusts his or her position. The mattress should feel comfortable not only when you fall asleep but when you awaken. If you wake up with back or neck pain, your mattress may not be providing proper support. Go bed shopping together to make sure that the mattress you select works for both of you. A good bed is well worth the investment.

Splurge on the best sheets you can afford with the highest thread count possible. They will make getting into bed feel special. Make sure that the temperature in your bedroom is not so warm that you are inhibited from nestling with your partner.

On most nights, couples should try to go to bed at the same time and adhere to the same sleep schedule. Even if one of you has to get up earlier than the other, you should still try to go to bed and wake up at the same time if it's possible. Couples should get into bed one hour PRIOR to the time they want to be asleep. So if you get up at seven in the morning and need eight hours of sleep to feel good the next day, you and your spouse should be in your bedroom by ten at night. The first forty-five to sixty minutes in the bedroom should be reserved for nonsleep activities, which might include cuddling, talking, or sex. If it's been a rough day, you can do some quiet meditation or stress-reduction exercises together. This hour should be about escaping from the rest of your life and being together alone in your bedroom, where you can maintain your special, intimate relationship.

No matter what happens in your life, you should guard and protect that hour. There may be times when one of you may be so restless that he or she needs to sleep in another room. But at least you will have an hour together to stay in touch, physically and emotionally, before actually trying to sleep.

If there are times when you can't sleep in the same room, try to set up an equally comfortable alternative sleep area. According to a recent article in the *New York Times*, the latest trend in new construction is the addition of a snoring room off the master bedroom so that "rather than endure elbowing or banishment to the den," snorers can sleep comfortably in their own space in the master suite. Of course, not everyone has the space or resources to so this, but you can still try to create a comfortable second sleep area by investing in a good bed, sleep sofa, or futon. Make the area an attractive alternative to the bedroom by using equally nice linens and blankets. Don't forget to include a music player, a reading lamp, and a small table for personal items. You don't want to make the other person feel as if he or she is sleeping in a less desirable outpost somewhere in the house. Both partners should feel equally comfortable and good about their sleeping areas.

## IF YOU HAVE TROUBLE SLEEPING

If you have persistent sleep problems that can't be solved by making lifestyle changes, you have two options. First, you can try one of several supplements to promote sleep that are sold over the counter. Second, you can check with your doctor about prescription medication.

Generally, we tell our patients to try the over-the-counter aids first. Melatonin supplements can be purchased at most natural food stores and pharmacies and are effective in inducing sleep in many people. We recommend taking 3 to 6 milligrams of melatonin before bedtime. Melatonin is sold in 1-milligram tablets, so we are prescribing a relatively high dose. We base this dose on our clinical experience and numerous studies on melatonin and sleep. The downside of melatonin is that at these high doses, many people find that they are still sleepy in the morning and well into the day. You need to try it and see how it works for you. Along with melatonin, we also recommend the mineral magnesium, sometimes called nature's tranquilizer. Both of these have a calming effect on the body.

If that approach doesn't work for you, there are several herbs that are good for inducing sleep. They include passion flower, valerian, hops, skullcap, chamomile, and gotu kola. Try to find a combination formula that includes several of these herbs.

If your sleeping problems continue, consider taking a prescription sleep aid medication. The new sleep aids are light years ahead of the old kinds that may have induced sleep but did not necessarily make you feel rested in the morning. The older generation of sedative-hypnotics (the benzodiazepines), such as Valium, Halcion, Klonopin, and Dalmane, worked on the central nervous system, specifically by exerting some effect on gamma-aminobutyric acid (GABA), a major inhibitory chemical in the central nervous system. Moreover, these drugs were often habit forming. There are several different types of sleep medications, and you need to take the right one for your problem. If your problem is that you have difficulty falling asleep, you should use a short-acting drug. If the problem is that you can't stay asleep, or you wake up too early, you need to use a longer-acting (medium length) medication. If you are taking any other medications, you need to consider potential drug interactions.

Below is some information about commonly prescribed sleep aids that may help you have a more informed conversation with your physician.

## ROZEREM

Rozerem is a melatonin agonist, which means that it binds to the same cell receptors as melatonin and behaves like melatonin. So why not just take melatonin? Rozerem may be more efficient and predictable than melatonin. Similarly to melatonin, Rozerem helps readjust your body clock to restore your normal sleep-wake cycles. Rozerem is the first prescription sleep aid that is not classified as a controlled substance because it does not work on the central nervous system and is not addictive. It has the fewest side effects of any of the sleep drugs. Although Rozerem works well for some of our patients, we have found that it doesn't work for everyone, specifically people who have taken sleep aids that have a more depressant effect on the central nervous system. If you're taking fluvoxamine, a drug most often given for obsessive-compulsive disorders, or have severe liver problems, you shouldn't use Rozerem. And, as with any sleep aid, you should not combine it with alcohol.

## AMBIEN

When it was first brought to market, Ambien and Ambien CR (extended release) were touted as vast improvements over the older sedative-hypnotic drugs. Although Ambien also works on GABA, it is far more specific than the other drugs, resulting in fewer side effects. It also clears out of the system faster, which means you're more likely to wake up feeling refreshed and not groggy. Despite some of its good points, there have been reports of Ambien causing some strange behaviors, including "sleep driving"—people getting into their cars while not realizing they were still asleep. We've prescribed Ambien to many patients with no adverse results, but nevertheless we caution people to be very careful with this drug, especially when they first start to use it. The effect of Ambien peaks within four hours after taking it; the drug is completely eliminated from the system within eight hours. Ambien is a good choice for people who have difficulty falling asleep and staying asleep.

## SONATA

Sonata is another newer drug that is particularly useful for people who have difficulty falling asleep. It usually induces sleep in about thirty minutes, and it can be taken late at night because it clears from your system very quickly. It's the only prescription sleep aid you can take if you don't have a full eight hours to sleep that won't leave you groggy in the morning. We recommend Sonata to patients who may wake up at two or three in the morning and have difficulty falling back to sleep.

## LUNESTA

Lunesta is another drug of choice for people who have difficulty falling asleep and staying asleep. Studies show that unlike the old sedative-type drugs, Lunesta doesn't disrupt normal sleep cycles, so it produces a more natural form of sleep. Most people tell us that they wake up feeling refreshed, as opposed to feeling as if they are coming off a heavy sedative. The downside is that you need to be able to devote eight full hours to sleep, or this drug will not clear from your system by morning.

# PART THREE

# YOUR GREAT LIFE MAKEOVER

## CHAPTER SIX

# SEX MAKEOVER

You've turned to this chapter because your sex life isn't what you think it should be, or what you and/or your partner want it to be. Maybe you've noticed that since you've hit midlife, things have changed in the bedroom—and not for the better. Or maybe you're pretty happy with how things are going but believe that there's always room for improvement.

The truth is, when it comes to sex, most midlife couples can use a tune-up. If you're concerned that your sex life is on the skids, if you feel that you or your partner are just not interested in sex anymore, if you're worried that one or both of you are not enjoying sex the way you should, the Sex Makeover is just what the doctor ordered.

When they have problems with their sex lives, people often have a nagging sense that something is wrong, but they're unable to voice their concerns. We're often surprised at how many men and women fail to make the connection between their physical problems and any emotional difficulties they may be experiencing. For example, it's not unusual for a man who is reluctant to have sex because of his erection problems to wonder out loud why he and his wife are growing apart. On the flip side, it's not unusual for a woman who's been struggling with bad menopausal symptoms to admit that she's lost interest in sex, much to the distress of her husband, but she doesn't have a clue as to why.

The first step of the Sex Makeover is to identify the key trouble spots that may be affecting your sex life, whether they are physical, emotional, or, as often is the case, a combination of both. By the time a couple seeks counseling, sex may have become such an emotionally charged issue that neither of them is thinking clearly. We engage the couple in a simple visual exercise to help break the ice. We draw a square and divide it into four quadrants: Her Physical Problems, His Physical Problems; Her Lack of Interest in Sex, His Lack of Interest in Sex. We then ask both members of the couple to pick out which quadrant best applies to them.

| Her Physical Problems | His Physical Problems |
|---|---|
| Her Lack of Interest in Sex | His Lack of Interest in Sex |

We have found that this simple device helps couples focus on what may be happening to one or both of them. For some couples, this exercise can be a true revelation. For the first time, a man may realize that it's not that his wife doesn't care about him anymore but that menopausal changes are affecting how she feels. And for the first time, a wife may realize that her husband would like to have sex with her but is afraid that he can't perform.

The second step is to solve any physical impediments that may be preventing a couple from engaging in sex.

The third step is to reestablish intimacy with your partner so that you both can begin to enjoy sex again.

We designed the following self-assessment quiz to help you pinpoint the areas in your life in which you may need help. We've divided the quiz into three categories: Sexual Health, Mood Matters, and Relationship Issues. When you finish the quiz, turn to page 90 to see what your answers may say about you and your relationship, and how the Sex Makeover can help you.

## DO YOU NEED A SEX MAKEOVER?

### SEXUAL HEALTH

*For Men*

1. Do you typically wake up in the morning with an erection?
2. Do you have more- or less-frequent sexual fantasies?
3. Can you usually masturbate to completion?
4. Are you losing muscle mass even though you haven't changed your activity level?
5. Have you recently started taking any new medication?

*For Women*

1. Are you ever bothered by vaginal dryness?
2. Do you have more- or less-frequent sexual fantasies?
3. Do you ever experience pain when you have sexual intercourse?

4. Are you having perimenopausal symptoms (like hot flashes)?

5. Have you recently started taking any new medication?

## MOOD MATTERS

1. Are you worrying more than usual?

2. Are you having increased difficulty with sleep?

3. Are you more irritable than usual? Are you having difficulty tolerating others?

4. Do you usually work more than nine hours a day, or more than five days a week?

5. Do you often clench your jaw or grind your teeth?

6. Do you feel tense most of the time?

## RELATIONSHIP ISSUES

1. Are you often angry with your spouse?

2. Do you ever feel disgust toward your spouse?

3. When you think about your spouse, do you notice any unpleasant feelings in your body?

4. Do you often worry that you will not perform well in bed?

5. Do you worry about your spouse's performance and/or physical limitations?

6. Do you find your spouse attractive?

## Understanding Your Answers

### SEXUAL HEALTH FOR MEN

**Question 1**

Most men wake up with a morning erection and have three or four erections while they sleep, primarily during REM, or dream, sleep. If you have morning erections or awaken at night with an erection, it's a good indication that your erectile function is intact. It doesn't mean that you can get hard and stay hard every time you want to have sex, but it rules out most organic problems as a cause of erectile dysfunction (ED).

If you never wake up with an erection, however, it's a sign of ED possibly due to poor blood flow, low testosterone, or nerve damage from an illness such as diabetes. (If you wake up at night with an erection due to a full bladder, it is not an indication of erectile function.)

About 40% of all men who are forty years old have erectile problems, and the number increases with age. If you're one of them, check out our protocol for treating ED on page 97.

**Question 2**

Sexual fantasies show that you have a healthy interest in sex. If a man doesn't have sexual fantasies, it's a sign of low libido, which is an indication of testosterone deficiency, excess stress, or even depression.

**Question 3**

If you can maintain an erection long enough to masturbate to completion, it's another sign that you are physically capable of having sex. If you find that you are unable to stay hard when you try to have sex with your partner, you may have other problems interfering with sex, such as performance anxiety, excess stress at work, or problems in your relationship.

If you can't stay hard long enough to masturbate, it could be a sign of a physical problem.

**Question 4**

When loss of muscle mass can't be attributed to a decrease in physical activity, it may be caused by lower-than-normal testosterone levels. Other symptoms of low testosterone include low libido, lack of energy, and erection difficulties.

**Question 5**

It's surprising how often doctors fail to tell their patients that the drugs they are prescribing could wreak havoc with their sex lives! If your sexual problems coincide with the new drug you've just started, chances are it's not mere coincidence and it's not your imagination. Once again, we refer you to the list of sex-busting prescription drugs for men on page 31.

## SEXUAL HEALTH FOR WOMEN

### Question 1

Vaginal dryness, a common side effect of estrogen loss, is one of the top reasons why women stop enjoying sex. Many of them don't even realize it! If you don't have proper lubrication, sex can be downright uncomfortable if not painful. Moreover, vaginal dryness can make you prone to chronic irritation and infection, which can put you in a very bad mood. There are many ways to treat this problem, and there is absolutely no reason why any woman should suffer from vaginal dryness. For more details, see "Her Sex Makeover" on page 106.

### Question 2

As with men, if a woman doesn't have sexual fantasies, it could be a sign of hormonal imbalance, specifically low testosterone, or it could also be due to excess stress or depression. Very often, it could be a combination of all three.

### Question 3

If something hurts, you try to avoid it. Sounds simple, right? You'd be surprised how many of our patients fail to realize that their desire to avoid sex is due to physical changes that make sex painful. If you answered yes to this question, we urge you to read "Her Sex Makeover."

### Question 4

From their mid-40s on, many women begin to experience perimenopausal symptoms, including sleep disturbances, moodiness, and irregular periods, that can be very disruptive. If these symptoms are severe enough, they can have a negative impact on all aspects of your life, including your sex life.

### Question 5

The medicine that you're taking to lower your blood pressure, treat your depression, or relieve your allergy symptoms could be disrupting your libido or interfering with vaginal lubrication. (Check the list of sex-busting prescription drugs for women on page 14.) If this is the case, you should talk to your doctor about switching medication.

## MOOD MATTERS

### Question 1

Many high-functioning people who outwardly appear as if they're taking everything in stride are walking around beset with anxiety and worry. What's worse is that they don't even realize it. They may be dealing simultaneously with tension at home, work-related issues, and health problems and believe that they're handling it all with equanimity, when in fact it's eating them alive. Stress has a way of creeping up on you and insidiously wearing you down bit by bit, both physically and emotionally. Not surprisingly, if you're in stress mode, your brain and your body are not focused on sex. What's surprising is how few people make the connection between their stressed-out state and their troubled sex life. The reality is, you really can't get it up if you're feeling down (see Chapter 3, "When You're Feeling Down").

### Question 2

Sleep is absolutely vital to your physical and emotional health in more ways than just the obvious exhaustion factor. Of course, if you don't get enough sleep, you'll be cranky, tired, and not able to function at your peak. But chronic sleep deprivation can disrupt normal hormone production, which can aggravate midlife hormonal changes. For women, sleep problems are typically linked to perimenopause, especially the decline in progesterone. Similarly, in men, the drop in testosterone can also trigger sleep problems. It can also weaken your immune system, raise your blood pressure, and increase your risk for obesity and metabolic syndrome.

For both sexes, insomnia is a classic sign of depression—and a loss of libido is one of the most common signs of depression. Even if you're not clinically depressed, waking up too early and not being able to fall back to sleep is often an indication that you are under excess stress.

Not sleeping is very *un*sexy.

### Question 3

When we ask patients whether they have been less tolerant of loved ones, friends, or co-workers than usual, those who say yes are typically genuinely surprised by their answer. People often don't realize that they've been short-tempered with others until they are forced to reflect on their behavior. Obviously, this can have a detrimental impact on their relationship with their spouses or partners. You don't need to be a psychiatrist to know that hurt feelings aren't conducive to a warm relationship. But if you don't realize how your behavior may be affecting others, you may not understand why your spouse is suddenly standoffish, and why you haven't had sex in weeks.

Irritability is also a classic symptom of perimenopause, for good reason. Women who are tired, stressed out, and generally feeling lousy are not going to be in the best of moods. What is lesser known is that the drop in testosterone can affect many men the same way. In fact, irritability can be a sign of testosterone deficiency.

**Question 4**

This is another question that often takes people by surprise. They don't realize that working long hours without enough down time can exact a steep toll on a midlife body. It's certainly an indication of not having enough balance in your life. Sure, you may have gotten away with all work and little play when you were in your 20s and 30s, but once you hit midlife, you need to take off time to recharge. (The upside is that you're smarter and can do things more efficiently!) This may not be true for everybody, but if you are feeling stressed out, and in particular you're experiencing changes in your sex life, you should rethink your work schedule.

**Question 5**

We've had patients who are absolutely confident that they're handling stress well, yet they answer yes to this question. If you grind your teeth in your sleep, or walk around with a clenched jaw during the day, you're showing telltale signs of a body under excess stress. Very often, you don't even know you're doing it until your dentist notices that you're wearing down the enamel on your teeth, or you're experiencing tension headaches or pain around your jaw line. You need to find better outlets for your stress. Even if you're unaware of it (or are in denial), it is undoubtedly interfering with other aspects of your life.

## RELATIONSHIP ISSUES

### Question 1

Unresolved anger toward your spouse is bad for your relationship and *terrible* for your sex life. To enjoy sex, you must feel safe and at ease with your partner. This is especially true for women. When there is anger or resentment, it can challenge your sense of safety and trust toward the other. In addition, there can be an internal conflict with engaging in an activity that brings pleasure to the person with whom you are angry. When anger festers, it only creates problems that compound steadily with time.

### Question 2

When people admit that they feel disgust toward their partner, we view it as a sign of a serious, often long-standing problem in a relationship. It is often a result of unresolved anger. Disgust could be a result of a change in physical appearance, such as weight gain, or circumstance, such as loss of employment or change in social status. Loving relationships can weather difficulties; fragile relationships often fall apart. If you have these feelings toward your spouse, it's a sign you need couples' counseling.

### Question 3

When you think of your spouse, what's your gut reaction? If you experience an uneasy feeling, you need to figure out why. The first and most obvious reason is that you may have some problems in the relationship. You'll know that better by how you answered the other questions in this category. If you said yes to the questions about anger or disgust, it's a red flag.

Even if you answered yes to this question, it doesn't mean that you and your spouse are on the rocks. Even people with loving relationships may feel queasy when they think of their spouses, but for entirely different reasons. For example, if your spouse has been ill, you may be literally worried sick about him or her. Or you may be concerned that your lack of sex drive or physical limitations may be adversely affecting your spouse.

### Question 4

Fear and anxiety are not conducive to good sex. If a couple has had difficulty with sex in the past because of a physical or emotional problem, it can haunt them well into the future, long after the problem has been resolved. Simply handing a man a bottle of Viagra is not going to erase his fear of failing again, just as giving a woman a vaginal lubricant is not going to completely ease her fears of pain during intercourse. Nor is it going to help reestablish the intimacy they may have lost, which is the foundation of a good sex life. Couples must first rebuild their relationship out of the bedroom before they feel comfortable again in bed.

### Question 5

Your spouse may be telling you in subtle ways—and not so subtle ways— that he or she wants to have sex, but you're holding back. Not that you don't want to, but you're concerned about your spouse. Maybe your husband has a heart problem and you're afraid that sex is too much for him (although his doctor says otherwise), or maybe the last few times, he wasn't able to get an erection and was so upset about it that you don't want to put him in that position again. Or maybe your wife has been complaining of arthritis and you're afraid that sex will hurt her, or you've noticed that she doesn't seem to be enjoying sex as much as she used to and you're worried that she's just doing it for you. All the while, your spouse may have no idea what's going through your head and may interpret your reluctance as rejection. You need to talk to each other in an open, nonthreatening, loving way. We direct you to "Honey, We've Got a Problem!" on page 113.

### Question 6

This can be a tough question for people to answer. People don't want to admit that they may not find their spouse attractive anymore, or that they can be so shallow that a few extra pounds or some wrinkles can turn them off. The truth is, when couples come to us to repair their relationship, they rarely feel this way. Happy couples tend not to focus on the negative; there's an expectation that there will be physical changes. A spouse in a good relationship will be more philosophical and say, "Yeah, we've both put on some weight, and maybe we don't look like we did when we were 25, but I still want to sleep with her (or him)." That said, engaging in the entire makeover as a couple, from diet to exercise, will make both of you feel livelier and sexier, which will translate into better sex.

A spouse who feels trapped in an unhappy marriage is going to be far more critical of his or her partner's appearance, as it is often a sign of deeper problems in the relationship. This type of problem requires consultation with a professional therapist.

## SEX MAKEOVER FOR MEN

When a midlife man seeks our help because he's worried about his sexual performance, the first thing we do is reassure him that he's not alone. Even though there is more frank discussion about sexual problems today than ever before, it's still very difficult for a man to admit that he's having problems in bed.

We've successfully treated men who have had problems for years before seeking help. When we ask them why they waited so long, they explain that they thought they were just "tired," or were not sufficiently aroused, or just weren't in the mood. The last thing they wanted to believe was that they had a physical problem impeding their sexual function.

Some men are so embarrassed—and sometimes ashamed—of their loss of sexual function that they'll sit in our office and talk about everything else until they finally admit why they came. Despite their outward bravado, men can be even more sensitive than women on some subjects—and their sexual prowess is one of them.

These men are comforted to hear that we see guys like them every day. We can tell them in all honesty, "This is no big deal. The reason Pfizer's stock went through the roof when Viagra came out was because there are so many men in exactly your position. The fortunate thing is that there are good treatment options now, and you can still have a great sex life, even if it hasn't been so good in recent years."

We encourage these men to talk to their wives or partners about their treatment, just to make sure that they're on the same page. Most women are happy that their husbands or boyfriends are asking for help, and they are relieved that the problem is out in the open. Some women, however, for reasons of their own, physical or emotional, may not be too interested in resuming their sex life. Their concerns need to be addressed as well, or sexual problems could persist for the couple even when the man no longer has any physical impediments.

**Our primary goal is to restore sexual function, not to mask the problem with drugs.** As detailed in Chapter 2, "The Hard Truth About Sex for Him," sexual desire and performance are closely linked to a man's lifestyle and overall physical condition. We can prescribe an ED drug to promote erections, but if a man is tired, is disinterested in sex, or has suffered neurological damage due to diabetes, he is not going to have a satisfactory sexual experience. In that same chapter, we review our comprehensive medical approach to diagnosing ED, which includes standard laboratory tests, hormone level checks, and other medical tests we may deem necessary, depending on the patient's history.

Based on the lab results, our patient's symptoms, and his medical history, we devise our method of treatment. Our first-line intervention includes dietary changes, weight loss, stress reduction, and supplements. If these simple interventions don't work, we turn to our second-line intervention: testosterone replacement therapy if needed and/or prescription medication for ED.

Our comprehensive approach will restore sexual function for most men, but not all. In severe cases, a man may not respond to treatment and may need more aggressive intervention, such as penile injections or a surgical penile implant. We refer these men to urologists for further treatment, and in most cases they, too, are able to resume sexual activity.

If a man is motivated enough to do what it takes, most sex problems can be successfully resolved.

## Rebalancing Hormones

If test results reveal that a man is severely deficient in testosterone, we prescribe hormone replacement therapy (HRT) along with lifestyle changes and supplements. If his testosterone deficiency is mild to moderate, we may try other interventions before resorting to HRT. (See "His Hormone Makeover" on page 201.)

We encourage everyone to eat their veggies, but it's especially critical for men who have elevated estrogen to load up on cruciferous vegetables, such as broccoli, cauliflower, Brussels sprouts, and cabbage. These vegetables contain indole-3-carbinol, a chemical that naturally blocks the enzyme in fat that converts testosterone into estrogen. Indole-3-carbinol can be destroyed during cooking; therefore, these vegetables should be eaten raw or very lightly steamed. We urge men to eat at least four to six half-cup servings per week. When we show men their lab results and explain to them that they may be able to improve them by eating more of these vegetables, even former broccoli haters find a way to love these vegetables! (Adding a pinch of sea salt to cruciferous vegetables can make them more palatable to people who don't like them.) We also directly supplement with indole-3-carbinol or its bioactive form, DIM. Our Web site, www.greatlifemakeover.com, has ongoing updates on the best products for supplementation.

Weight loss—especially around the abdomen—can help reduce estrogen in men and pump up testosterone. That beer belly is full of fat cells that make estrogen out of an enzyme called aromatase. Get rid of the beer belly, and you've gotten rid of a sizable amount of unwanted estrogen.

We also recommend three supplements to tame estrogen—either diindoylmethane (DIM) or indole-3-carbinol, calcium-D-glucarate, and resveratrol (see page 100)—to help men control estrogen conversion and indirectly give their testosterone levels a mild boost. Pro athletes and body builders, who want to preserve every micromole of testosterone they make, use these same supplements. You'll find brands designed just for guys in the sports supplement section of health food stores. If estrogen conversion is occurring at a rate that cannot be reversed by supplements and dietary changes alone, we may also prescribe an estrogen blocker, Arimidex or a similar drug, which usually works well.

### Get a Handle on Stress

Excess stress—specifically chronically high levels of stress hormones circulating throughout your body—can disrupt the production of sex hormones and wreak havoc on your sex life. If your sympathetic nervous system is in overdrive, your body is primarily concerned with survival. Your adrenal glands are pumping out cortisol to get you ready to fight or flee, and they are not attending to their other job: producing sex hormones. That means that the parasympathetic nervous system, which relaxes smooth muscle and is essential for an erection, can't do its job.

The reverse is also true. Sexual problems can be so upsetting that they rev up your production of stress hormones at the expense of your sex hormones. Stress may or may not be the primary cause of your sex problem, but if you don't get a handle on it, it can certainly make the problem worse.

We refer you to Chapter 11, "Mood Makeover," to help get you back in the mood.

For men, several studies have shown that regular exercise significantly reduces the incidence of erectile dysfunction. According to a major study involving 31,742 male health care professionals, ages fifty-three to ninety-three, "Lifestyle factors most strongly associated with erectile dysfunctional were physical activity and leanness." The study suggested that burning at least 200 calories a day through some type of physical activity could help protect sexual function. That's really not so hard to do. It's as simple as taking a brisk walk for thirty minutes, swimming for about twenty minutes, lifting weights for thirty minutes, or riding your bike (stationary or outdoor) for thirty minutes. If you do more vigorous exercise, such as take a spinning class, you can burn 200 calories in about fifteen minutes.

## PRESCRIPTION DRUGS FOR ERECTILE DYSFUNCTION

The lifestyle interventions that we recommend, such as improving your diet, losing weight, and getting more exercise, will definitely help recharge your sex life, but it could take a while for the benefits to kick in. In some cases, even if a man does everything we tell him, he may still need additional help. If he is testosterone deficient, we supplement him with prescription testosterone, which often does the trick for all andropausal symptoms, including ED. However, sometimes even when testosterone is replaced or is not deficient to begin with, and the other makeover plan is initiated, a man may still not get the desired result. In these situations, we prescribe one of the three drugs approved by the Food and Drug Administration to treat erectile dysfunction: Viagra (sildenafil), Levitra (vardenafil), or Cialis (tadalafil).

All three drugs work by inhibiting an enzyme, phosphodiesterase type 5 (PDE-5), which is concentrated in penile erectile tissue, blood platelets, and smooth muscle of the blood vessels, and which interferes with a man's ability to have an erection. An erection is a well-choreographed event that involves a few key players in the vascular and nervous systems. Nitric oxide (NO) is one of them; it is a colorless gas produced by many cells in the body that controls the muscular tone of blood vessels and is essential for perceiving pleasure and pain. NO stimulates the production of guanylate cyclase to produce cyclic guanosine monophosphate (cGMP), which causes the relaxation of corpus cavernosum smooth muscle that is critical for an erection.

PDE-5 inhibitors can make an erection physically possible for men who may not be able to have one otherwise. Please note, however, that these drugs are not aphrodisiacs. They don't rev up sex drive or make a man want to have sex. A man must be sexually aroused for these drugs to work in the first place. If a man is low in testosterone, is depressed, or has little interest in sex, these pills may not do a thing.

## Is This ED Drug Really Necessary?

Before we prescribe an ED drug, we talk to our patients to make sure that they really need one to have a satisfactory sex life. A man may not be able to get as strong or hard an erection as he used to, but he may still be able to enjoy sex, albeit differently than when he was younger. He may require more manual or oral stimulation from his partner to get aroused and stay aroused. He may need to find new ways to bring his partner to orgasm by means other than intercourse, such as manual or oral stimulation. Sexual aids, such as vibrators (which can be used on men and women) or penile rings (a vibrating ring worn around the penis) can be useful in terms of making sex exciting—and playful—for both partners (see page 111). Very often, women are fine with this and may even like it better, particularly those who are experiencing vaginal thinning and enjoy extra foreplay. A couple may resolve these problems by making simple changes in how they make love and may never require drug intervention.

What a man may lack in hardness can be offset by experience and technique. Women respond to men who are caring lovers, not necessarily the biggest studs. Teenage boys are not exactly known for their lovemaking skills, despite the fact that erections come quickly and easily to them. If you let it, your age and experience can work for you here.

On the other hand, we've encountered couples who are very clear that halfway isn't good enough. We recently treated a healthy 60-year-old man who was dating a 35-year-old woman, and he was concerned about his inability to get completely hard while having sex. We understood his feelings and prescribed Viagra, although he probably really didn't need it to complete sexual intercourse, but he definitely couldn't sustain as strong an erection without it, and he felt more confident and satisfied with it.

## When Drugs Don't Work

Despite the hype surrounding them, these drugs don't work for everybody. About a third of men who try an ED drug don't have a satisfactory result and simply give up. Some men are very disappointed because they don't get an erection after the first try. A minority may find the side effects intolerable. The usual side effects are headache, blurry vision, or stomach upset; in most cases they're mild, but for some men they can be severe.

So why don't ED drugs work for all men? Part of the problem may be that some of these men are relying solely on these drugs to fix their erectile dysfunction and not doing anything else to improve their health. In our experience, men who also adapt positive lifestyle changes fare the best on these drugs. The first and most obvious reason is that these men are helping to improve blood flow to the penis on their own, which means they're relying less on the drug.

The second reason is not so obvious and is one that is often forgotten by both physicians and patients. A drug is only as effective as the body allows it to be. By that we mean that when you take a drug, your body still has to metabolize it; drugs taken orally are broken down by the liver, where they are detoxified. Metabolism is supported by good nutrition. Someone who is eating well, living a healthful lifestyle, and avoiding toxins is going to be a better metabolizer and have fewer side effects with these and other medications.

Third, not every drug works well for every man. The first drug you try may not work for you or may have an unpleasant side effect, but the second drug—or even the third drug—you try may be fine. Sometimes it's a matter of simply adjusting the dose. It's important not to get discouraged and to keep trying until you get the desired result.

These drugs work best when prescribed as part of an overall treatment plan that considers the complete biology and psychology of the male reproductive system. These drugs can't repair a fragile relationship or restore sexual confidence on their own. Performance anxiety on the part of the man or the couple can interfere with sex even if the problems have been resolved. We urge all men who are starting an ED drug to read over "Honey, We've Got a Problem!" on page 113. Popping a pill is not going to erase months or even years of miscommunication or hurt feelings in a troubled relationship.

Although most men can use ED drugs safely, some cannot. These drugs are not to be used by men taking any form of nitrates for chest pain, or alpha-blockers for high blood pressure. When taken with those drugs, PDE-5 inhibitors can cause a sudden and dangerous drop in blood pressure. With all ED drugs, there is also a small risk of priapism, a prolonged erection in which blood fails to drain from the penis. This can be quite painful, requiring a visit to the emergency room.

## Which ED Drug Is for You?

From a medical perspective, all ED drugs are basically the same, with slight variations. None of these drugs produces an instant erection; they take about half an hour to become effective. We encourage men to give the drug up to an hour to take full effect. This allows a more relaxed approach, and given that they all last for at least a few hours, there is no need to rush. Some couples actually like having the extra time to get cozy and romantic.

Viagra and Levitra last up to 4 hours. Cialis can work up to 36 hours, which means that it stays in your system longer. This is better if you want spontaneous sex, but it could be worse in terms of potential side effects. If a couple loves spontaneity, then Cialis is a good choice. If they don't mind planning for sex (which isn't a bad idea), then the other drugs are fine. We often recommend that a man bring his wife or partner with him to his doctor's appointment so they can discuss these options. It's also important for a couple to establish early on that even if a man takes an ED drug in preparation for sex, if his partner doesn't want sex at that time, she shouldn't be coerced into it. These drugs should be used to enhance a relationship, not to put a strain on it.

Launched in 1998, Viagra is the oldest ED drug and the one we've been prescribing the longest. Unless the patient or his partner has a strong preference otherwise, we tend to prescribe it first. If it doesn't do the trick or has an annoying side effect, we increase the dose and see if it is more effective. In many cases, the higher dose will work, but if it doesn't, we then switch to another drug to see if it works better. For reasons we don't fully understand, despite the fact that these drugs are pretty similar in how they work, some men do better on one than on another.

In clinical studies, Viagra has been proved to be effective in ED that results from spinal cord injuries and antidepressant medications. It doesn't mean that the others are not similarly effective, just that clinical data for these uses are not yet available.

Fatty food interferes with the absorption of Viagra, which works best on an empty stomach. Try to plan your meals at least 2 or 3 hours before a sexual encounter. Unlike sildenafil (Viagra) and vardenafil (Levitra), peak serum concentrations of tadalafil (Cialis) are not affected by a high-fat meal.

### Beyond ED Drugs

Fortunately, there are usually other solutions for these men, such as penile injections or implants. They're not as convenient or easy as taking a pill, but they work well for many men. You can find out more about these treatments from a urologist.

## PENILE INJECTIONS

In pre-Viagra days, penile injections were hailed as a real breakthrough in the treatment of ED. They're still a good option for men who can't use the drugs. Using a very fine needle, a man injects medication into the base of his penis, which results in an erection usually within 15 minutes or less. The erection typically lasts for up to 2 hours. Unlike ED drugs, these injected drugs will produce an erection without sexual arousal. The most commonly used drugs are pavaparine hydrochloride, phentolamine (Regitine), and alprostadil, a synthetic form of prostaglandin E1 (Caverject).

Obviously, some men are squeamish at the mere thought of giving themselves a shot in an area as sensitive as the penis, but the reward of a satisfying sexual experience is enough to help men overcome their fears. There is always a risk, albeit a small one, of injury and infection. As with ED drugs, there is also a small risk of priapism, a prolonged erection in which blood fails to drain from the penis, which can be quite painful.

## PENILE IMPLANTS

If all else fails, a penile implant can take over the erection function of the penis. The most popular is the internal penile pump, which consists of two silicone-covered expandable cylinders that are implanted into the corpora cavernosa of the penis. The cylinders are connected by tubing to a separate reservoir of solution implanted in the groin muscles. A pump is implanted under the scrotal sac and connected to the system. To produce an erection, you press down on the pump, thereby forcing the fluid into the cylinders. When you no longer want an erection, you can press a release valve on the pump and deflate the cylinders. The inflatable implants have a very high success rate and offer hope to men who may have no other option.

## PRACTICE SAFE SEX

Women who have not had a period for a year are considered to be postmenopausal and do not need to use birth control. This is great news for women and their partners, as long as they're in monogamous relationships with people who are free of any sexually transmitted diseases. If you're not in a monogamous relationship, or if you're having sex with a partner who may have contracted an infection in the past, you need to use a latex condom at all times—and that's whether you're having vaginal sex, oral sex, or anal sex. Latex condoms are considered highly effective against HIV (the cause of AIDS) and gonorrhea, and they substantially reduce the risk against chlamydial infection. Although condoms do not offer 100% protection against all sexually transmitted diseases, they substantially reduce the risk for many of them. Of course, you still need to exercise caution when selecting your partners.

# HER SEX MAKEOVER

The two most common sexual symptoms we hear from women are decreased libido and discomfort when having sex. Hormonal shifts during menopause can sap a woman of her interest in sex, regardless of how happy she may be in her relationship. If a woman has lost her desire for sex, we recommend a check of her hormone levels to see if she is testosterone deficient. Hormone replacement therapy (HRT) can be very helpful in these situations. However, as we'll discuss later, if a woman doesn't feel happy and secure in her relationship, all the testosterone in the world may not motivate her to engage in sexual activity. For women, the psychological aspects of sex are every bit as important as the physical aspects—and possibly even more important.

We address both the physical and the emotional aspects of sex to restore sexual function.

## Getting Her Comfortable with Sex

The most common physical complaint among women is vaginal dryness and thinning, which can make sex very uncomfortable. Fortunately, with so many women reaching menopause these days, there are numerous over-the-counter products, including vaginal lubricants and massage creams to restore moisture and enhance sexual pleasure. Many are sold right at your local pharmacies and discount drug stores, in specialty stores, through catalogues, and on the internet. A once taboo subject, vaginal lubricants are now advertised on television!

There are many lubricants to choose from. Some are to be used daily, and other "sexual enhancers" are for use during intercourse. The lubricants designed specifically for sexual activity tend to be somewhat heavier and thicker than the normal lubricants, which helps provide a slick surface to avoid friction. These are probably not products that you want to use every day.

Many women need to use a lubricant every day or so to maintain surface moisture and avoid chronic irritation. It's best to avoid petroleum-based products (those containing mineral oil) because they can disrupt the normal flora of the vagina as well as interfere with the effectiveness of a condom. If you have sensitive skin, always try a small amount of the cream or gel on the outside skin of your vagina before rubbing it on the delicate inside tissues. Leave it on for 24 hours. If it causes any irritation, don't use it again! Steer clear of products with preservatives like parabens, which can be irritating. Our patients report that Replens, Sylk (made from the kiwi fruit), K-Y Jelly, and Senselle work well for them, but not all brands work for everyone. If one product is irritating or doesn't do the job for you, try another.

If over-the-counter products don't do the trick, we prescribe a vaginal estrogen cream, which many women find to be very helpful. Estrogen vaginal cream is considered safe for most women because very little actually gets absorbed into the body. In addition, women with severe symptoms should consider hormonal rebalancing with HRT, even if it's just for a short time to get them through a rough patch. If you're not sleeping well or suffer from vaginal dryness, or if sex hurts, you're not going to be too interested in pursuing romantic encounters

Our patients tell us that one sexual enhancer, a massage oil called Zestra Feminine Arousal Fluid, works very well if applied to the clitoris, labia, and vaginal opening prior to intercourse. This herbal-based nonhormonal product increases blood flow to the pelvic area, stimulating sexual response and lubrication. (Their partners like it, too!)

Extra foreplay can also help increase lubrication naturally. After menopause, it may take a bit longer for the vagina to become lubricated than it did before, so build in some extra time for sex.

And don't forget about the "G" spot, the highly sensitive area 2 to 3 inches inside a woman's vagina on the top of the vaginal wall. Gently stroking the "G" spot from the outside of the vagina can be very pleasurable. It's good to alternate between touching the clitoris and the "G" spot because too much stimulation of the clitoris can actually make it feel numb. Some vibrators are designed for "G" spot stimulation, and some women prefer them to conventional vibrators.

## Is It Time for a Change?

If sex is not enjoyable or is even painful, a change of position can also make it more comfortable and pleasurable for women. What might have been an erotic sexual position for a woman before she had children or became menopausal may actually be uncomfortable for her now.

For example, the standard missionary position (the man stretched out on top of the woman) may put too much pressure on a woman's legs and genital area, which can make a woman tense and tighten up. And that just makes sex even more painful. It is also a bad position for people with arthritic hips and knees. A better choice is a modified version of the missionary position, in which a woman fully bends her knees, with her legs open and relaxed. A pillow placed under the woman's hips can relieve pressure.

If lying down is too much of a strain for either of you, try having sex in a chair, with the woman on top, either facing the man or facing outward for rear-entry position. (Just make sure it's a sturdy chair and won't topple over. Imagine explaining that one to the neighbors!)

Lying side by side, facing each other, is another joint-friendly position that takes pressure off the pelvic area and is enjoyable for many women.

Rear-entry positions also work better for some women who find the front entry to be uncomfortable.

Consider other forms of sex. Many couples find that oral sex can be very pleasurable even if a woman has vaginal thinning or dryness.

The point is this. Just because what worked in the past doesn't work anymore doesn't mean that it's time to throw in the towel. Experiment with different positions to find one or more that makes sex pleasurable for the two of you. Do things to please each other.

Many women tell us that the good thing about midlife is that they are more confident than when they were younger, and they are better able to express themselves on a sexual level. Don't be afraid to ask for what you need and want.

And remember, sex is supposed to be fun. Trying out new positions may feel strange, but don't be afraid to laugh about it together and to have a good time, even if it doesn't always work out.

## Emotional Comfort

Being physically fit and hormonally balanced are key issues for the midlife woman. Although we don't want to confirm stereotypes, for women, the state of the relationship is critical to their willingness to engage in sex, so, the psychological aspect of sex is often more important to a woman's sexual functioning than it is for men.

There is a strong connection between a woman's feelings about her partner and sexual desire. A 2006 study, conducted by researchers at the University of Michigan of 3,300 women nearing menopause, found that greater sexual desire was "more strongly associated" with the state of a woman's current relationship and the availability of a sexual partner.

We have found this to be the case among our patients. Those who are happy with their partners are more eager to have sex with them and more willing to take the necessary steps to correct any problems that may be impeding their sexual relationship. We've had women say to us, "I'm not as interested in sex as I used to be, but my husband wants it, and I like it because it's a way for us to be close."

For a woman, feeling comfortable with her partner is fundamental to good sex. We carefully evaluate this aspect of the equation for women (not that we ignore it for men), because comfort with one's partner is crucial. If unresolved resentment has settled in the relationship, it can lead to physical revulsion on a woman's part. This is especially the case if there has been some violation of trust. You have to be turned on to have sex, and that's not going to happen if a woman's partner psychologically and emotionally turns her off.

For example, we recently saw one couple, Pam and Bill, who were having problems in the bedroom despite the fact that they would describe themselves as basically a happily married couple. When Bill approached Pam for sex, she would almost recoil, and when she reluctantly agreed to have sex, it wasn't enjoyable. Pam initially told us that their problems began when Bill bought their 18-year-old daughter a sports car after the two of them agreed that they would not get her a car because of safety and other issues. But after a few sessions with the couple, we learned that Pam had long believed that Bill frequently made important decisions unilaterally, often against her wishes, and, in fact, he had. The purchase of the sports car was the tipping point that brought her resentments to a head. Pam was furious at Bill, and she needed to have it out with him until he really heard her, responded sincerely, and attempted to make amends. Most of all, he needed to become a more collaborative partner in his marriage. After a few sessions of relationship coaching, during which they really learned how to talk to each other, their sex life restarted.

Although not all situations can be resolved as easily as this one, if a woman can be assertive in talking things out with her partner, she will have a better sexual and overall relationship. When unresolved anger is allowed to fester, it can affect everything in a relationship, especially sex.

We have seen some women in bad relationships, who think they will never enjoy sex again, find that they can have great sex in a new relationship. The saying "I never thought I would be able to feel this way again" has a biological reality to it.

This doesn't mean that if the spark is gone, you should ditch him and go on the hunt for someone new. Unless there is extreme dysfunction in the relationship, things usually can and should be resolved. It does mean, however, that trying to make a bad relationship better is worth the time and trouble.

Sometimes the problem is one of familiarity through lots of years of being together. This can cause both members of the couple to get lazy in the romance department. Doing some romantic things together as if it's a new relationship can make all the difference in the world.

Low libido that is accompanied by other perimenopausal or menopausal symptoms requires a hormone assessment.

## Sexual Aids Can Help, Too

When it comes to using sexual aids, the times are changing—for the better. *Newsweek* recently reported that vaginal vibrators, lubricants, vibrating penile rings, and other products are now being sold in big chain stores like Walgreen's, CVS, and even Wal-Mart. This reflects not only a more open attitude toward sex but the fact that a growing number of baby-boomers are turning to these products to jump-start their sex lives. Sexual aids are also sold in "respectable" catalogues and Web sites with products geared for midlife women, from companies with such conventional names as Time for Me, As We Change, and Too Timid.

Sexual aids can be very useful in providing some extra help for men and women who need it. They can also be fun, and add some variety and zest to long-term relationships where familiarity may make sex less exciting.

Many couples use sexually oriented videos to get turned on. This is fine, but keep in mind that male and female views of sexuality can conflict when it comes to pornography. Hard-core porn tends to turn women off, even if some men like it. Women tend to prefer the more sensual, albeit sexually explicit, videos that have romantic plots. We also recommend watching tantric sex instructional videos together. Tantric sex is loosely based on a blend of Eastern philosophy and the Kama Sutra. Although these videos can be explicit, they are not offensive to women in that they emphasize good sex in terms of a warm, loving relationship.

In addition to revving up sexual desire, many of these videos give a few pointers on better sex. If you do an internet search for "tantric sex" you will find numerous Web sites offering instructional materials for couples.

It's important that both members of the couple feel comfortable about using sexual aids. It's not a good idea to ambush your partner one night with a new gadget that he or she may not want or like. Nor do you want your partner to think that he or she isn't stimulating enough, so that you have to resort to exotic devices. How, then, do you bring up this subject in a way that won't offend or scare off your partner? A woman or man could say to his or her partner, "I was looking through this catalogue and saw something I thought would be fun for both of us." If her partner pursues the topic, she can even show it to him. Many men might find this to be intriguing.

A man could say to his wife, "I know it takes a bit more to get both of us going these days when we have sex. I was wondering if next time you'd like it if we used a vibrator?"

After using a sex aid, partners should be sure that they both enjoyed it. Ask your partner, "How was that for you?" or "Was that a good amount of pressure?" or "Should we try that toy again?" or "Would you like to try that in a different position?" It's important to understand that you may not get it right for both of you the first time, so you can have some fun trying again . . . and again.

## EXERCISE IS AN APHRODISIAC

We can't overstate the importance of maintaining a fit body during this period of life, when many women begin to gain weight and lose confidence. Regular exercise helps control many of the symptoms of menopause that contribute to sexual problems. A study conducted at the University of British Columbia found that 20 minutes of intense exercise revved up a woman's interest in sex. In fact, sexual response seemed to peak around 15 minutes after a workout. This is another good reason why we recommend that couples work out together. There are several reasons why exercise may prove to be an aphrodisiac for both men and women. In the short run, vigorous exercise triggers the release of endorphins, the feel-good hormones in the brain that contribute to an overall feeling of well-being. That certainly can put you in the mood. Furthermore, exercise relieves stress and activates the parasympathetic nervous system, which sends blood flow to the genitals. In contrast, the sympathetic system, which gets the body ready for flight or fight, directs blood flow to your legs to allow you to run fast. When you're in flight or fight mode, you are thinking about survival, not sex.

## HONEY, WE'VE GOT A PROBLEM!

In discussions about sex, even the best of couples have difficulty saying what they're actually thinking. Very often, one partner completely misinterprets how the other really feels. It may sound like a cliché to say that good sex comes down to communication, but it's absolutely true. We spend a great deal of our time teaching couples how to talk to each other, particularly how to bring up these sensitive issues without alienating their partners.

Before we go any farther, you need to know the Number One rule for getting your relationship back on track. Don't sound as if you're accusing your spouse of being neglectful, insensitive, disinterested, or whatever else you may think he or she is. Instead, talk about how YOU feel, using the word "I" instead of the accusatory "You." "I'm upset that we're not the way we used to be." "I miss the time we used to spend together." It's a lot less threatening than saying in so many words, "It's all your fault!"

We hate to perpetuate stereotypes, but sometimes even the most well-meaning of men can really be rather dense when they begin to express themselves on this topic. Sometimes we literally have to put the right words in their mouths.

A case in point is our 53-year-old patient Larry, who came in for counseling because his wife, Karen, no longer wanted to have sex. She never actually said that she didn't, but he noticed that whenever he made an overture to her, she became snappish and critical. Larry had noticed a few other things, too: Karen used to wear sexy nightgowns to bed, and she now wore his pajama tops. She had gained a few pounds during the past year and was having problems sleeping. Not an insensitive man, Larry wondered if his wife could be going through some menopausal issues that were making her feel bad about herself. Larry's solution was to try to reassure his wife that he loved her by trying to be more physically affectionate, but that only made her even more standoffish. Until the past year or so, the couple had had a pretty good sex life, so Larry was upset—and frustrated—by the downturn in sexual activity and by what he felt was the deterioration of a good marriage.

This is a time when many men need a crash course in how to talk to the women in their lives. We are often surprised by how men can be rather unprepared when it comes to articulating a supportive statement that will resonate with—and not alienate—the women they love. This way of talking is very foreign to most men, and they need to work at it. We explained to Larry how menopause can affect a woman's physical and emotional health. We raised the issue that Karen not only could be feeling badly about her appearance but could actually be experiencing physical symptoms that could be making sex uncomfortable. And rather than risk putting herself in a vulnerable position where he might say to her, "Sex isn't good anymore," she was simply avoiding it.

After explaining to Larry all the issues that his wife could be struggling with, we asked him to express what he wanted to say to her to reestablish communication. Larry did what a lot of men tend to do. He shifted into his logical, left-brain way of thinking, trying to bring the problem to a quick resolution. He replied, "Honey, you need to stop being so self-conscious so we can start having sex again."

## Left Brain to Right Brain

Larry's heart was in the right place, but his approach needed some finessing. We explained that although a man may want to rush through the emotional discussion and get right to the solution, that's not what his wife wants or needs to hear. Rather, he needs to appeal to his wife's right brain, the emotional center, which is struggling tremendously (and often needlessly) with the changes of aging.

We focus on teaching men a few key concepts that are tried and true and that have worked well in the past. In a nutshell, here's some advice we give men on how to effectively express their feelings to the women they love.

Reinforce your love for your wife or partner and your desire to be close to her—with the caveat that it must be true. We know that many men are uncomfortable expressing emotions, and the language we recommend may seem excessive or extreme, but in reality it's not. We ask a man, "Do you love your wife and are you still attracted to her?"

Assuming the answer is yes, we then suggest that he try saying, "I might not be good at telling you enough, but I hope you know that I'm still madly in love with you and very much attracted to you physically." It's often difficult to get a man to say these words out loud, because to him they sound over the top. But that's because men tend to think that their wives really know how they feel, when in fact they don't. They need to hear the words.

He then needs to explain what's on his mind in a direct, clear way: "I feel like we have grown distant in some ways, and I don't want that."

Sometimes it can be disarming for a man to ask his wife, "Are you feeling okay with me?" If she brings up her own insecurities about changes in her body, this is an opportunity for him to reassure her that they are not a big deal for him, although he appreciates that they may be a big deal to her.

At times, a wife may admit that she may not be as attracted to her husband as she once was, either because he has gained weight or because he has been sloppy about his dress and overall grooming. If the relationship is strong, however, a change in physical appearance doesn't usually make that big a difference in terms of sexual attraction. Nevertheless, a woman likes to feel that a man has a high enough regard for her to put some effort into his appearance, both when he's at home and when they're going out.

Perhaps even more important to women is a belief that their partners are *true* partners, not just when they're in bed but in their everyday lives as well. Men tend to forget that women are often torn in many different directions, having to juggle work with managing a household while tending to the needs of children and older parents. For many women, the "second shift" begins when they get home at night. By the time they've finished making dinner, cleaning up, and doing other chores, many women are exhausted and do not necessarily feel amorous. Men often underestimate the importance of pitching in and being a good helpmate around the house. A recent study reported that men who share in the housework have more frequent sex and more satisfying sex lives than men who do not. This is not surprising: A woman who feels that her partner understands the challenges of her life, and that he is there for her, is going to feel more romantically inclined than a woman who is resentful over her partner's lack of participation.

Acknowledge where you have been at fault in not maintaining intimacy, and don't be defensive about issues she brings up about you. This is not a competition to prove who's right or wrong but must be viewed as an opportunity to patch whatever series of mismatches have occurred in your interactions.

Nonsexual affection can be very helpful during this type of conversion. Sit close to your wife and put your arm around her, but don't make any moves that suggest your prime motivation is to get her into bed.

Don't try to solve your problems then and there, which is the default mode for many men. Very often, what a woman needs most at this time is to be listened to.

Compliment all the positive things she brings to the relationship. Compliments are free, yet we never cease to be amazed at how stingy people are with them.

The problem-solving should be a joint brainstorming session in which you carefully listen to what she has to say and discuss possible strategies. Let her know you want to work with her. You need to work together as a team.

Reinforce that this is not about sex per se—as much as you enjoy having sex with her—but about closeness and intimacy, of which sex is an important component.

Men come back and tell us that that they wished they had learned to talk to their wives like that decades ago. The positive response they get from their wives diminishes the lack of control they were feeling in the situation—a feeling nobody likes to have (especially men!).

## What's on His Mind?

Susan, 49 years old, bright and attractive, came to our Center ostensibly because she was interested in our HRT program. But, as we later learned, something else was weighing heavily on her mind. In the course of our discussion, she commented that she thought that her husband, Mark, 52, could benefit from our program as well. When we asked her why, she told us that in the past year her husband had changed, and not for the better. He seemed more tired and irritable than usual, and he showed absolutely no interest in sex. In fact, the couple had not had sex within the past six months, and the last few times they had tried to have sex, Mark was very upset that he couldn't get an erection. When Susan tactfully tried to bring up the subject of sex, Mark simply shut down, as men in his position are apt to do.

Susan observed that until then, the couple had had a good sex life, and she didn't understand why he wouldn't talk to her about it.

"We're too young for this!" Susan said. "I don't want to be in a sexless marriage for the rest of my life. Is there anything you can do for us?"

The first thing we did was reassure Susan that she wasn't alone, that there were many couples in similar situations. It sounded to us as if her husband had a physical problem that was interfering with his ability to maintain an erection. And if he was like most of the men we see in our practice, he was absolutely devastated by it. We explained to Susan that for many men, self-esteem is closely tied to masculinity, virility, and potency. Mark might have been thinking that Susan would think less of him if she knew that he was having sexual difficulties. He might not even have accepted that he had a problem in his own head. He might be dismissing his sexual problems with "I'm tired" or "I'm not in the mood right now." Like many men in his situation, he was hoping that the problem would just go away on its own.

Susan was very comforted by our explanation. Even in the best of marriages, a wife may understand intellectually that her husband has a problem, but on an emotional level, she may interpret his behavior as a personal rejection. It's not uncommon for a woman to think, "He isn't attracted to me anymore" or "It must be those 5 pounds I've put on recently" or even "He's seeing somebody else." That's why we urge men to talk to their partners honestly about their sexual difficulties—but of course, that's easier said than done.

We knew that we could do a lot to help Mark, but first we needed to get him into the office for a full evaluation. We coached Susan about how she should approach her husband about getting him into treatment without making him defensive.

## Right Brain to Left Brain

In these cases, we have found that men respond well when information is presented in a factual, nonemotional way. When a woman mentions this subject to her husband, she should appeal to his left brain and be overt: "I've noticed some differences the last time we had sex, and I'm concerned about your health. Erectile changes can be associated with medical problems, and I want you to go to your doctor to have things checked out. I'd like to go along if it's okay with you, because I care about you. If it turns out to be simple erectile dysfunction associated with a midlife body, then there are some great treatment options to discuss with the doctor."

Another good approach is to disarm the man by taking the onus off him. Try saying, "I've noticed that we haven't had sex recently, and I really miss it. Is there something I'm doing that's making it difficult or uncomfortable for you? Am I less approachable than I used to be?" This gives a man a chance to open up and admit he's having a problem. Although many men will be relieved to finally bring the subject out in the open, others may still be reticent. Don't accept a brush-off as an answer. Stay calm, but be persistent.

It's important to end the discussion with an action plan that gets followed up. Perhaps the next day one of you will call the doctor for an appointment for a checkup. Or you'll promise each other to pick up the conversation where you left off. And then do it!

In some cases, a man may acknowledge that he can still get an erection but has occasional difficulty, and is very worried that he'll perform poorly when he's trying to have sex. You can reassure him that you enjoy being close to him even if sex doesn't always work out every time, and that there are ways that you both can have a satisfying experience without intercourse. Simply knowing that he's not expected to perform in a specific way can help him better cope with his anxiety.

## RESTORING INTIMACY: STEP BY STEP

One or both members of the couple may have had physical problems that interfered with their sexual enjoyment, or maybe the couple has simply drifted apart, consumed by work or family obligations. We may have successfully treated their physical and emotional barriers to sex, but they still have a lingering anxiety about resuming sexual relations. If sex has been physically painful for a woman, just the mere thought of sex can trigger intense fear. If a man has had erection difficulties, he may feel very nervous that it's going to happen again, even though he is now perfectly capable of maintaining an erection, thanks to lifestyle changes and/or medication. The memory of a few awkward experiences or false starts can make a couple shy away from sex. The last thing they need is to perpetuate a cycle of failure by jumping in too strongly or too soon before one or both of them are ready.

The first and most important step is to reestablish intimacy. The couple needs the trust and warm feelings that are the foundation of good sex. Couples need to take a step backward to get to know each other again in the context of a romantic relationship. We help couples design a specific program to get them back in synch, physically and emotionally. Couples who are working this through on their own can adapt some of these techniques in their own relationship.

We recommend that couples set aside one or two nights a week as date nights. We also recommend that they *not* have sex during the first month—that's right: no sex. By taking sex off the table, the couple can relax with each other without worrying about how they're going to perform. We work out a schedule in which the couple starts off slowly and over time works up to intercourse.

We suggest that couples begin with a romantic dinner, at home or out, with the understanding that at the end of the evening they can hug and kiss, maybe even cuddle in bed. But they know ahead of time that they don't have sex, even if they think they might want to. We don't want either partner worrying that sex is a possibility because it could make him or her hold back.

On the next few dates, the couple goes a bit farther in terms of resuming physical contact. Perhaps they give each other a gentle massage with some nice essential oil, or take a bubble bath together, and then end the evening by cuddling in bed. Touching in this way can be very intimate—and again, no matter how erotic it might feel, the understanding is that they do not proceed to sex.

The program sets loose goals for each date so that they steadily move forward until they are both absolutely comfortable with each other. The point is to get the couple in the mode of touching each other and being romantic with each other without the sex. Then they gradually allow more and more sexual contact. Eventually, they take it to the point where sex is optional. After the first month, if they want to proceed to full intercourse, great. If they don't, that's fine, too.

We encourage couples to do physical activities that are not related to sex to get their bodies back in touch with each other. Working out together is a great way to regain physical confidence as individuals and as a couple. Taking a ballroom dancing class and swimming together, for example, are good physical activities that promote closeness.

After you've resumed sexual activity, you need to incorporate intimacy into your lifestyle. Many couples find that scheduling a date night or two during the week works well for them. We know that many couples like being spontaneous, but if you leave sex to chance, it may never happen. Or it could take one of you off guard when you're not ready.

The upside is that you can plan for sex and look forward to it. Planning ahead can allow a couple to carve out more meaningful time together to prepare the bedroom for a romantic evening. One important caveat is this: you must have an understanding that date night doesn't always culminate in sex if one partner doesn't want it. The point is not to put more pressure on each other, but to enjoy good quality time together.

## CHAPTER SEVEN

# DIET MAKEOVER

The right diet can help you achieve a trim, strong body; enhance your sex life; and boost your mood. If you want to look better and feel better, you have to eat better. In creating the Diet Makeover, we want to show you how to make the best food choices for your health.

Our diet helps restore hormone balance, enhances metabolism, improves blood flow (so important for male and female sexual response), and boosts mood. The diet is an extraordinarily potent tool for regaining health, energy, and sexual function in men and women.

We both eat a plant-based diet—one that is rich in vegetables, some fruit and whole grains—but we each do it differently. Dr. Bazzan is a true vegan: he avoids all animal products. Dr. Monti eats a plant-based, low-sugar diet but with modest amounts of lean animal protein, especially fresh fish. We offer sample menus that include all vegetarian meals, or meals with animal protein. The choice is yours.

## FOR A HEALTHY RELATIONSHIP

Try to sit down and have at least one meal daily with your partner. Make it an enjoyable experience. Shop together, cook together, and make that meal time a social experience.

Some of you may be wondering: If I don't eat meat, how will I get enough protein? The truth is that there are excellent plant sources of protein, including legumes (beans), soy, and whole grains. Furthermore, if you want to include some animal protein in your diet, it's fine. But it has to be the *leanest* protein, primarily fresh fish or white-meat chicken or turkey.

In our experience, well-informed patients make the best choices. There is strong scientific evidence to support our dietary principles, which we'll discuss here. By the end of the Diet Makeover, we hope you'll be convinced of the merits of eating a plant-based diet. We urge you to try the diet for at least 3 weeks. At the end of those 3 weeks, we know that you'll love how you look and feel. You will be lighter, healthier, and more energetic. Many of our patients are so thrilled with the results that they stay on our eating plan forever.

## BETTER FOOD CHOICES FOR BETTER SEX

The typical American diet is an inflammatory nightmare. As we have discussed earlier, chronic inflammation is considered an underlying causative factor in both long-term chronic disease (like heart disease, cancer, diabetes, and asthma) and short-term illness.

Ideally, a healthful diet not only provides necessary nutrients but also creates an alkaline (versus acidic) body pH, which decreases inflammatory factors in the system. Acid-producing foods include sugars, simple starches, red meat, and animal fat—the mainstay of the typical American diet. Alkaline-producing foods are many vegetables, especially the green leafy ones; some whole grains; and some fruits.

Most Americans do not eat enough vegetables and fruits. That's a fact. A large study published in the *American Journal of Preventive Medicine* in 2007 showed that despite the launch of a national fruit and vegetable campaign in 1991, the dietary intake of vegetables and fruits by Americans did not show an increase between 1999 and 2002! Only 27% of adults in the United States consumed three or more servings of vegetables per day; 29% consumed two or more servings of fruit as recommended by the USDA; but only 9% met both guidelines!

## Too Much Animal Fat Is Bad

One of the most remarkably consistent findings in studies about dietary intake for humans and other mammals alike is how destructive animal fat is to our health. Study after study implicates dietary animal fat in heart disease, stroke, high blood pressure, high cholesterol, diabetes, and many cancers, including breast, prostate, and colon cancer, to name just a few. Which foods contain this saturated animal fat? Red meat and full-fat dairy products. (Not only is the fat in dairy products problematic but they contain a type of protein that may promote cancer, which we'll discuss later.)

Harvard researchers have linked animal fat to an increased risk of colon cancer. These findings have made their way into the media, but obviously not far enough into the consciousness of Americans to stop them from consuming so much meat and high-fat dairy products such as cheese and cream. For men, dietary fat from animals has been linked to prostate cancer. In yet another recent Harvard study, researchers found that men who ate large amounts of animal fat were 1.79 times more likely to develop advanced prostate cancer than were men who ate less fat.

Women take note: In 2004, researchers reported strong evidence that fatty acids derived from the diet may play an important role in the origin and progression of breast cancer. Also, a very recent study showed that a high intake of meat, particularly processed meat, increased the risk of premenopausal breast cancer.

Men take note—before you bite into that "manly" steak, think about this: In 1990, a study at the University of Utah School of Medicine offered the first documentation, to the researchers' knowledge, of the "acute effect" that a fat-containing meal has on testosterone levels. They found that a fat-containing meal reduces testosterone concentrations, indicating that fatty acids may actually have an effect on how much testosterone is produced by the testes. They found that men who drank a liquid made with nonnutritive sweetener, or who ate a meal combining carbohydrate, protein, and minimal fat, did not show a reduction in testosterone.

Two years later, researchers at Ball State University in Indiana noted that testosterone concentrations decreased significantly after a fat-rich meal. In their study, they found that one hour after men ate a meal rich in animal fat, total testosterone levels were decreased by 22%, and free testosterone (the bioactive testosterone circulating throughout the body at the time of the test) was 23% lower. And these levels remained significantly low for eight hours. In addition, men who are fat, especially in the midline, typically have lower testosterone levels.

Furthermore, we know that poor blood circulation is the leading cause of ED—and that is a direct result of heart disease and diabetes, two epidemics caused by a high-sugar diet loaded with bad fat.

The evidence supporting this—and supporting the fact that dietary animal fat is harmful—is irrefutable.

## Trans Fats Are Really Bad, Too

You find the other bad fat—trans fat—in margarine, fried foods, and many baked goods and processed ready-to-serve foods. Historically, trans fats have been added to foods to increase their shelf life and to enhance the stability of oils used for frying, like hydrogenated oil in shortening. They still make up about 2% to 3% of total fat intake in the United States. Butter contains a small amount of trans fat, but margarines not modified to reduce trans fats may contain up to 15% trans fat by weight.

More recently, some cities—New York for one—have gone so far as to legislatively ban the use of trans fats in foods that restaurants prepare. Fast food giants

Wendy's and KFC made headlines when they announced they would no longer use trans fats in cooking or preparing french fries; Taco Bell and McDonald's later announced they would follow suit.

Trans fats are bad because they interfere with the normal function of our cells and create inflammation. Thus, they are more likely to create both cell damage and arterial plaque formation, leading to cardiovascular disease. Plaque can cause injury to the arterial wall, which can rupture and cause the formation of a blood clot, which can block blood flow to the heart.

Both saturated fat and trans fat have also been shown to promote inflammation. Conversely, the good fats are in fatty fish (like salmon) as well as in plant-based foods: flaxseeds, avocados, nuts, and vegetable oils (olive, canola, and nut and seed oils, such as sesame), and they appear to bestow anti-inflammatory properties. Since inflammation is part of the disease process, foods with anti-inflammatory properties, logically, are also disease-fighting substances.

In early 2006, three major reports from the Women's Health Initiative (WHI) were issued, generating a great deal of discussion and controversy. The Women's Health Initiative was a major fifteen-year research program involving 161,808 women. It was begun by the National Institutes of Health (NIH) in 1991 to address the most common causes of death, disability, and poor quality of life in postmenopausal women: cardiovascular disease, cancer, and osteoporosis.

The reports indicated that reducing total dietary fat over an eight-year period did not lower the woman's risk of heart disease, specifically coronary artery disease. Nor did this reduction appear to lower the risk for breast or colon cancer in postmenopausal American women. But how could this be?

The answer is actually pretty simple. When the researchers measured total dietary fat, they did not distinguish between bad fats (saturated fat and trans fatty acids) and good ones. Back in 1991, as you may remember, we were told to eat a "low-fat" diet as a cure-all. Later we realized that very low fat was actually unhealthful. But we now know, as we discuss in this chapter, that just as the bad fats are harmful, the good fats—such as omega-3s, part of the family of the polyunsaturated fatty acids, otherwise known as PUFAs (found in salmon, flaxseeds, and walnuts) and mono-unsaturated fats (found in vegetable oils and in almonds, Brazil nuts, cashews, sesame seeds. and pumpkin seeds)—are crucial to the health of the body. Just remember that cell membranes are made of a layer of water sandwiched between two layers of fat. So no fat is not an option, bad fat creates problems, and the right fat is indispensable.

| MONO-UNSATURATED FAT CONCENTRATIONS IN PLANT-BASED FOODS | |
|---|---|
| | SOURCE% MONO-UNSATURATED FAT |
| Olive oil | 73 |
| Canola (rapeseed) oil | 60 |
| Hazelnuts | 50 |
| Almonds | 35 |
| Brazil nuts | 26 |
| Cashews | 28 |
| Avocado | 12 |
| Sesame seeds | 20 |
| Pumpkin seeds | 16 |

Since the researchers neglected to discern between the good fats and the bad fats, their findings about risk for disease were not meaningful.

## Bad for Your Bones and Metabolism

Not only does excess animal-based protein put you at risk for life-threatening diseases, but it also, oddly enough, breaks down the strength of your bones. It turns out that the strong advice to drink milk when we were kids should have come with the adage to stop drinking it when we become adults. Both the protein and the fat in milk are problematic for many people. For others, the sugar (lactose) is a big problem. In addition, it is rather allergenic and can be inflammatory and mucus-producing. We recommend that adults get their calcium from other sources, such as green leafy vegetables.

Instead of drinking milk, the real way to preserve bone may be by *reducing* your intake of animal protein. The Harvard Nurses' Health Study, which observed some 85,000 nurses (female and male) for twelve years, yielded some fascinating findings about calcium leaching from the bones. The researchers found that the people who ate a diet high in animal protein had a significantly increased risk of breaking their forearms. The risks were highest for women, and in those who ate even one serving of red meat a day, the risk for fracture was higher than in women who did not eat a serving a day of red meat. Additional studies have linked the consumption of meat protein with increased risk of fracturing a hip. Of course, you need still to eat adequate protein, but you don't have to rely on red meat. There are many excellent vegetable sources of protein in addition to fish and lean poultry. Sure, you can have a steak on occasion if you want one (choose the leanest cuts, please!), but you shouldn't make it the mainstay of your diet.

Moreover, dairy protein may be carcinogenic; researchers found that cancerous tumors in rats grew well when the rats were fed more than 10% of their diets in the form of casein, a protein that is the heart of dairy products. Conversely, when rats were given more than 20% of their diets in the form of plant protein (soy, nuts, legumes, beans) or only 5% in animal protein, the tumors failed to grow at all. We don't know for sure whether this is true for humans, but it's alarming enough that we advise our patients to steer clear of casein.

## THE CHINA STUDY

*The China Study* hit the shelves in the form of a book late in 2006 and quickly became a best seller. Researcher and author Dr. T. Colin Campbell subtitled his book *The Most Comprehensive Study of Nutrition Ever Conducted and the Startling*

*Implications for Diet, Weight Loss and Long-Term Health.* Although there are always limitations to an epidemiologic study, and the results cannot be considered conclusive, his work suggests some rather remarkable findings. People in China who ate the most animal-based foods got the most chronic disease. People who ate the most plant-based foods were the healthiest and tended to avoid chronic disease.

How did Dr. Campbell determine this? Well, it took twenty years to complete, and involved about 6,500 participants from 65 counties and 130 villages in rural mainland China. Dr. Campbell chose villages in rural China because the people there eat less than half the fat as do other regions, as well as about three times the amount of fiber. Moreover, in these villages, only about 10% of the protein eaten comes from animal sources, and the total cholesterol of these residents averaged around 127 mg/dL, versus 203 mg/dL for the same population (adults ages 20 to 74) in the United States.

Dr. Campbell's team analyzed information on some fifty diseases, including seven different cancers, by collecting blood, urine, food samples, and detailed information on food intake from the participants. He was astounded over the clarity of the results. Dr. Campbell found that for both men and women in China, the villages with diets higher in green vegetables and sources of mono-unsaturated fatty acids had lower risk of death resulting from coronary artery disease. Likewise, the more salt found in their urine and apolipoprotein B found in their blood, the higher was their risk of death resulting from coronary artery disease. Apolipoprotein B proteins are found in the blood of people who eat meat. The more frequently the Chinese villagers ate meat, the higher was their risk for disease. The more frequently they ate plant-based proteins, legumes, and light-colored vegetables such as cauliflower, broccoli, and squash, the lower was their risk for disease. Simple as that. Our mothers were right. We should eat our vegetables. Later in this chapter we give you delicious recipes to show you how to cook these health-giving foods to preserve both their flavor and their nutrients.

## NATURAL, UNPROCESSED IS BEST

We've had more than one patient ask if eating an order of french fries counts as a serving of vegetables! They weren't kidding. Clearly, if they are prepared poorly, even vegetables can be bad for you. So here's what you need to know to make the right food choices.

Vegetables, fruits, and grains are all carbohydrates. Not all carbohydrates are good. In fact, we make a sharp distinction between "nature-made" carbs and processed "man-made" carbs.

"Nature-made" carbohydrates include vegetables, grains in their whole, unadulterated, nonprocessed form, and fruits. Overall and with few exceptions, foods in this category are safe to eat daily.

"Man-made" carbohydrates include pastas, breads, chips, cookies, and other processed starches. These items start out as something in nature, like a wheat kernel, and get processed and adulterated to, say, a sticky bun or a snack food (not to mention all the bad fat in most of these items). Man-made carbs break down rapidly into simple sugars and burden the system with a high glucose load, contributing to diabetes and other problems when eaten too often and in portions too large. They are also highly inflammatory. We also want you to avoid simple sugars, such as refined table sugar and corn syrup, particularly high-fructose corn syrup, which is the primary ingredient in commercial sodas. This doesn't mean you can never indulge your sweet tooth; just do so only on special occasions.

---

### DIET TIP

Avoid "all or nothing" thinking. If you happen to eat a cookie at a party, don't tell yourself, "Now that I've blown it, I may as well just binge on bad things for the night." Nothing could be farther from the truth. When you deviate, surround the bad food with good, nutritive food. In fact, we believe that once you've been strictly on our diet for a few months, and assuming you are in a good state of health, you will have the reserves that will allow you to deviate once in a while and rebound just fine.

---

## ADDING SPICE TO LIFE AND HEALTH

We never cease to be amazed by the power of plant-based foods to contribute to human health. As it happens, some delicious spices also show some ability to reduce hunger, improve mood and brainpower, and even help muscles stay strong. Here are some of the highlights:

**RED PEPPER TO CURB HUNGER**
The *British Journal of Nutrition* published a study showing that when women added 2 teaspoons of dried red pepper to their food, they ate fewer calories during the meal.

**CAPSAICIN TO PUT YOU IN A GOOD MOOD (AND MAYBE IN THE MOOD)**
Capsaicin is the substance that adds the heat to chili peppers. It triggers pain receptors in the mouth, signaling your brain to rescue it by releasing endorphins to

make you feel better. As a result of this activity, the fire is eventually extinguished in your mouth, and you feel good, too. Not bad for a little spice.

## TURMERIC, A NATURAL ANTI-INFLAMMATORY

Turmeric and its main bioactive compound, curcumin, has the power to block inflammation and improve heart health. Natural plant polyphenols (flavonoids), such as epigallocatechin gallate, found in green tea, and curcumin, have been reported to have access to the brain and to possess multifunctional activities, such as metal chelation, free-radical scavenging, anti-inflammation, and neuro-protection.

Research has shown that turmeric can also help muscles repair themselves after heavy exercise. It's best to use the spice a few days before a major workout for the best effect.

## ROSEMARY FIGHTS FREE RADICALS

This fragrant herb contains high amount of antioxidants, which protect against the potentially damaging effects of free radicals. Free radicals are chemicals naturally produced by the body as part of normal energy production by our cells. In excess amounts, they can be harmful and have been linked to premature aging and to an increased risk for cancer and heart disease.

Want to keep fresh herbs on hand all the time? We recommend that people grow their own herb gardens. If you don't have a backyard, or live in a city, you can keep a few pots of different herbs on a balcony or shelf near the kitchen window. You can cut off a few sprigs every day to soak in your olive oil, sprinkle on salads, or put in your food.

### Eat Nuts!

Studies have shown that nuts, particularly walnuts, can have a positive impact on cardiovascular health. One recent study showed that men who snacked on nuts cut their risk of sudden death by heart attack by almost 50%. That's because nuts are high in omega-3 fatty mono-unsaturated fats that lower LDL, the bad cholesterol, and increase HDL, the good cholesterol. Having high levels of HDL helps keep coronary arteries nice and open and smooth, enabling oxygenated blood to flow freely to all parts of the cardiovascular system.

Other foods high in mono-unsaturated (lifesaving) fats include olive oil, canola oil, avocados, and flaxseeds. Although nuts are high in calories, research shows that the body probably doesn't absorb all the calories in nuts. Still, moderation—about a handful, which equals around an ounce—gives men the heart-protective benefits. Also, we recommend the health benefits of walnuts and almonds over peanuts, which can be highly allergenic and inflammatory for some. Also, be sure to eat them unsalted or very lightly salted. One tip would be to buy them unsalted and raw and to add a touch of sea salt or some of your favorite spices (see recipe for Dan's Trail Mix on page 145).

## Quinoa—the Super Grain with Protein

Quinoa (pronounced KEEN-wah) is a super grain that is not technically a grain. The seed contains all eight essential amino acids and is extremely nutritious, gluten free, and protein rich. Although quinoa is higher in unsaturated fats and lower in carbohydrates than most grains, it can be used in place of rice in cereals, main dishes, soups, side dishes, salads, and desserts. You can cook quinoa in very little time (less than half the time it takes to cook rice), and it contains calcium, iron, phosphorous, vitamin E, and lysine. Although it may sound like a food that has been designer-made for the twenty-first century, quinoa was found in South America several centuries ago. It's now grown and harvested in the Rocky Mountains.

To cook quinoa, rinse it thoroughly to remove the saponin, the sticky substance on the outer part of the grain. Saponin naturally repels birds and insects, so it is a useful quality of the seed. The ratio is about 2 or 3 cups of water to 1 cup of quinoa. After the water boils, reduce the heat and simmer until it's tender but not mushy. Enjoy it with some olive oil and chickpeas!

## Fresh Greens and Food Safety: How to Wash Leafy Greens

None of us will forget the frightening *E. coli* outbreak associated with fresh bagged spinach that killed three people and sent almost two hundred more to the hospital in 2006. These outbreaks are caused by poor hygiene and fecal contamination of the vegetables in the handling chain. This outbreak, and others in the recent past, have involved fresh leafy greens, especially lettuce, spinach, and sprouts. But unpasteurized juices are also a potential source of *E. coli* contamination, especially apple cider, because it's made from apples that have fallen off the tree (the *E. coli* is a contaminant from the ground) rather than those that need to be picked.

Many people are left scratching their heads as to whether or not it is safe to eat fresh leafy greens. The answer: yes and no. Yes, you should eat fresh produce and enjoy it. For some plants, the highest nutritional yield is in the raw form. But no, you should not be blasé about washing the greens. Wash all unpackaged produce under running water. You should even rinse off prewashed produce because it can still attract bacteria. Soaking produce is okay, but that doesn't take the place of washing it under running water as well.

The truth is that there is some unavoidable risk in eating fresh uncooked foods. That is true of organic produce as well, because all farming methods carry a risk of contamination from irrigation water tainted with cattle waste, contaminated flood water, or a problem in a processing plant, like the use of water for washing that hasn't been properly filtered or chlorinated. In addition, the foods that usually contain *E. coli* are not acidic, because the bacteria implicated in these outbreaks don't grow well in acid conditions. In the United States, it is up to the Food and Drug Administration to ensure the safety of the food that reaches our tables. But we can help by keeping kitchen counters, cutting boards, and utensils clean; washing our hands; and rinsing produce. If the minimal risk frightens you, cook your vegetables thoroughly at 160° F for at least 15 seconds. Unfortunately, doing so kills the enzymes in them.

## HIM

*"I had put on weight and was beginning to show early signs of Type 2 diabetes. I was a terrible eater—I just ate what I wanted without thinking about it. My usual lunch was a big hero sandwich stuffed with luncheon meat, a bag of potato chips, and few Cokes. I would*

*come home at night and curl up on the couch. I was too tired for anything. My wife convinced me to take steps to stay healthy so we don't have to spend our later years going from doctor to doctor. We did this together.*

*After seeing Drs. Bazzan and Monti, I knew I had to change the way I eat. I followed their advice and started eating a lot more fresh vegetables and whole-grain bread. My typical lunch these days is a lean turkey sandwich on whole wheat bread, and a side salad. I drink water or homemade ice tea. No more junk or sweet stuff. I have a piece of fruit for a snack. My diabetes is under control, and I feel great. Having a partner that you enjoy being with is wonderful. We want to travel together, continue to build our business, and enjoy each other's company. We're looking forward to our future together."*

### HER

*"Since menopause, I had gained about 10 pounds and was very unhappy about it. This was a good opportunity to change the way we eat so we would both get healthy and hopefully stay that way. I decided to become a vegetarian, at least to lose weight. I liked it so much that I'm still a vegetarian. I just feel better, and the weight came off so easily.*

*We both work, so we cook together at night. We both eat lots of grains and vegetables, but my husband sometimes adds some fish, lean meat, or chicken to his dinner. It's a good thing that we're doing this together. It makes it a lot easier."*

## GETTING STARTED

By now you know that you'll be eating a diet rich in vegetables, some fruits, whole grains, and lean protein. We provide a list of acceptable foods on page 148. For the next 3 weeks, design your meals from this list. After that, try to stick as closely as possible to the list to maintain your good results.

On page 150, we provide a week's worth of sample menus. These are to be used as guidelines, not to be followed slavishly. We don't expect you to eat food that you don't like. The food lists contain a wide enough variety to accommodate most palates.

## EAT THREE MEALS AND TWO SNACKS

In addition to breakfast, lunch, and dinner, eat one snack midmorning and one midafternoon. Try not to eat any food after seven in the evening.

## DIVIDE YOUR PLATE INTO FOUR QUARTERS

Fill three-quarters of your plate with vegetables. Fill the remaining quarter with your protein source or whole unprocessed grains (brown rice, quinoa, millet, etc.).

## DON'T EAT ANIMAL PROTEIN AND GRAIN AT THE SAME MEAL

Animal protein does not digest as easily with grains as it does with vegetables.

## DRINK WATER, HERBAL TEA, OR HOMEMADE VEGETABLE JUICE

Avoid soda, caffeinated beverages, alcohol, and commercial juices.

## NO MORE THAN TWO SERVINGS DAILY OF FRUIT

Stick to fruit choices that are highest in antioxidants (see list on page 149).

# FOR THREE WEEKS, VEGGIES ARE YOUR MAIN FOOD GROUP

Vegetables should constitute a large part of your diet. Strive for at least seven servings a day. **One serving is ½ cup of cooked vegetable.** You can eat unlimited amounts of most vegetables, especially green vegetables.

For the first three weeks, don't eat white potatoes or corn, and limit carrots to one serving per day. These vegetables are higher in simple carbohydrates and sugar.

Stick to fresh vegetables only; don't use canned or frozen. Cooked vegetables should be **steamed lightly**, lightly sautéed, or baked so they are tender but still crisp. Include large amounts of **green leafy vegetables** (spinach, romaine lettuce, kale, collards, chard) and choices from the **cabbage or cruciferous family** (cabbage, cauliflower, broccoli, Brussels sprouts).

Include some **orange, yellow, and red vegetables** (carrots, beets, squash, yams, red and yellow pepper, yellow corn).

Conventionally grown peppers, celery, green beans, and cucumbers are the most highly contaminated with pesticides. If you eat them, buy organic only.

Rinse all your vegetables very well to wash off germs and pesticide residue.

### You Can Drink Your Vegetables, Too

You can create fresh vegetable-juice cocktails that balance carrots with greens (kale, collards, etc.) and other low-carbohydrate vegetables (broccoli, celery, etc.). These should be *organic* vegetables. (Pure carrot juice is not recommended because of the high natural sugar content of carrots.) A vegetable cocktail is a great antioxidant-rich snack, but as good as it is, it's no substitute for eating several additional servings of whole vegetables daily. With vegetables, more is better!

### Sprouts

Sprouts are an excellent concentrated source of phytonutrients. Try mung bean, radish, alfalfa, and broccoli sprouts. Broccoli sprouts may be a bit harder to find than the others, they but contain many times the antioxidant value of broccoli. Sprouts are baby plants and full of energy. They deliver living energy to the body. People who introduce sprouts into their life always come back impressed by their power to improve health. Ask in your health food store for local people who grow them and sell them, or look on the internet.

# PROTEIN

**Eat minimal amounts of lean protein**. People need an adequate—but not excessive—amount of protein each day to maintain muscle mass and maintain proteins in the blood. **We generally recommend approximately two to four 3-ounce servings for women (6 to 12 ounces total) and three to six 3-ounce servings for men (9 to 18 ounces total).** Men and women with high activity levels may require more animal protein than those who are less active. Furthermore, if you need extra animal protein to fill you up, then by all means go for the higher amount.

The focus of your meal should be on vegetables and whole grains if you eat meat. Animal protein foods should take up no more than a quarter of your plate, with vegetables making up the remainder.

Fish and eggs whites should be your only source of animal protein for the initial three weeks. Legumes (beans) and soy foods are great vegetable protein sources. If you must eat chicken or turkey, be sure it is derived from free-range poultry raised without hormones or antibiotics. Red meat and organ meats should be avoided because they are too high in saturated fat and too inflammatory. You can begin to incorporate more animal protein into your diet after the first three weeks, but even then we prefer that red meat be excluded.

Preferred fish are cold-water, deep-ocean varieties such as white-fleshed fish, which are low in total fats. Some examples are cod, haddock, orange roughy, and sole. Also recommended are the fattier types such as bluefish, herring, mackerel, sablefish, salmon, and tuna (particularly albacore). These fish are excellent sources of omega-3 fatty acids, which help your body reduce inflammation, protect against heart disease, help inhibit cancer growth, and benefit the immune system. Because of potential contamination, fish such as tuna or swordfish should be limited to twice per month. Avoid farm-raised fish because they often contain high levels of chemical contaminants. Landlocked? It's easier than ever to purchase freshly frozen wild salmon, cod, tuna, and other varieties at health-conscious stores such as Trader Joe's and Whole Foods. The fish comes completely scaled and cleaned, and it can be easily thawed in a bowl of water. Buy a variety of fish and stock them in your freezer.

Soy-based products are now more prevalent than ever. We especially prefer tempeh (cultured soy) as a good protein source that contains all the essential amino acids and also provides iron and calcium. Also, there are numerous soy and tempeh preparations available that are quite tasty. Buy a few and experiment, and try some of the recipes offered. Be sure to check the labels and buy soy products that have not been genetically modified.

Soy yogurts are remarkably similar in taste to dairy-based ones. Get a brand and flavor that limits the sugar content to 10 grams or lower per serving—which should be a guiding principle with any sweetened food, even though you will now be eating foods with natural sweeteners. Natural things in excess can be bad, too. Soy yogurts will qualify in the snack category of our meal plans.

There are now some soy- and vegetable-based cheeses that can be used to enhance your meals, but be sure to read the labels. Some contain milk or casein, a potentially problematic milk protein.

## A Word About Phytoestrogens

Some foods, notably soy foods (tofu, tempeh, and soy milk) and flaxseeds contain chemicals that mimic the action of estrogens in the body. These foods are beneficial for both men and women—up to a point. There is some controversy as to whether excess soy foods can stimulate the growth of prostate tumors in men. Paradoxically, some studies show that soy foods can reduce the risk of prostate cancer. Since the science on this issue is confusing at best, we recommend that men limit their intake of phytoestrogenic foods like soy to 4 ounces per day.

Some women find that soy foods help relieve menopausal symptoms, such as hot flashes and night sweats. Although some studies suggest that soy is protective against breast cancer, there has been theoretical concern that the estrogen compounds in these foods could potentially fuel the growth of existing breast tumors. Overall, we feel that soy-based products are beneficial for women (unless they have had breast cancer, in which case the science is not yet clear and we do not recommend soy for now) and suggest a daily maximum of 4 to 6 ounces of soy foods per day.

# WHOLE GRAINS

Eat only whole, unprocessed grains. Avoid refined, polished, and processed foods such as pasta, rice, bread, crackers, and snack foods.

If you have any autoimmune problems such as rheumatoid arthritis, fibromyalgia, or psoriasis, avoid foods that contain gluten, which includes most grains. Brown rice is usually well tolerated, but be careful of the quantity if you are trying to lose weight. You can flavor your grains with whatever herbs you like (e.g., fresh parsley) or Bragg Liquid Aminos (a healthful alternative to soy sauce).

# PREPARING YOUR KITCHEN

We believe that when it comes to diet, the emphasis should be on adding and replacing, rather than taking away. That said, there are definitely some things that need to be minimized or eliminated. The diet won't feel overly depriving if done right, and it can be a fun bonding experience to prepare for it with your partner. The two categories below are *What to Put into Your Kitchen* and *What to Remove from Your Kitchen, Now.*

Clean your refrigerator as an initial preparatory step. Have the vegetable storage compartments sanitized and ready for use. Tidy your cupboards and counter spaces to create a pleasant, workable environment.

Plan times with your spouse when the two of you can go to the market—ideally, two times per week.

## What to Put into Your Kitchen
### SIMPLE THINGS TO HAVE READY IN YOUR KITCHEN
A large mixing bowl for salad preparation, sharpened knives, peeling utensil, juicer (optional), at least one cookware item with steaming capacity (e.g., pan with removable steam basket [All-Clad and Cuisinart cookware have nice ones]), steam apparatus (Black & Decker and others). If you don't already have a large basket or ceramic platter for your kitchen counter or table, get one so you can have your fresh vegetables and fruits proudly displayed and easily accessible. In it can go all the items that do not require refrigeration, such as zuc-

chini, tomatoes, lemons, apples, and avocados. This will give your kitchen a nice organic feeling while mentally connecting you to the vibrant foods you will be eating.

Buy vegetables that are easy to prepare. For example, many grocery stores now have prewashed, prepackaged salads and greens (remember, organic is best!). It is so easy to put the package in a bowl and add our simple dressing (see page 146 for recipe). For extra flavor and nutritional value, add some avocado, sprouts, onion, or whatever herbs you like.

## GOOD FATS: OILS, NUTS, AND SEEDS

Olive is the preferred oil for salads and cooking; canola is fine, too. Olive oil should be cold pressed and extra virgin to insure maximal health benefits. Buy a large glass bottle of it, and store it in a cool, dry place. Stock your kitchen with a variety of raw seeds and nuts: pumpkin seeds, sunflower seeds, sesame seeds, flaxseeds, walnuts, and almonds, but NOT peanuts (because of their high mold content), and only cashews that are raw and vacuum packed. Nuts should be purchased fresh and raw, and stored in the freezer. See our delicious snack recipes for nuts and seeds.

Seeds can also be pulverized in a grinder and sprinkled over soups, salads, and cereals. Flaxseeds are a rich source of essential fatty acids (omega-3) and are encouraged. Avocado, which is actually a fruit, provides an excellent and tasty source of fat. Buy three avocados a week, and use them in salads or to make guacamole.

### What to Remove from Your Kitchen, Now

- All dairy products, including milk, ice cream, butter, and milk-based yogurt. All bad fats, including margarine and commercial mayonnaise.
- Canned vegetables and canned fruit (give them to your local food drive).
- All sweets, including all cakes, candy, and cookies.
- White bread, commercial cereals, white pasta, white rice.

## MEAL PLANNING

We offer a week's worth of menus for men and women to provide a blueprint of how to put a day's worth of meals together. Don't feel compelled to follow these menus slavishly; they are meant to be suggestions.

Don't worry about portion sizes when it comes to fresh vegetables, especially leafy greens and sprouts. In fact, your plate of vegetables may look bigger than your old meals. That's okay. In fact, you sometimes need more than twice the volume of vegetables to equal half the calories of a denser processed food you used to eat. People rarely overeat fresh vegetables because their bodies know what to do with them and know when to send the signal that enough has been consumed, as opposed to processed foods such as simple sugars that jolt the body and create cravings.

### Breakfast Is a Must

People are often at a loss about breakfast when the goal is to have a predominantly plant-based diet. "If I can't have bacon and eggs, then I don't know what to eat." First, get out of the mindset that breakfast food has to be what you grew up on, or what is typical for this culture. If you've ever been to other countries, like Japan, you've seen some radically different approaches to breakfast. The important thing is to have a nutritious breakfast that is tasty.

Morning can be a great time to use your rice cooker or steamer to prepare a variety of grains. We like to combine several whole grains in a big jar (e.g., wheat berries, oat groats, quinoa, brown rice, amaranth) and simply pour them into the rice cooker to cook while we tend to the other activities of getting ready in the morning. When the grains are ready, we sprinkle on freshly ground flaxseeds (or whole seeds, though you may not extract the same value), mix in a few almonds or seeds, or sprinkle on a little of any flavoring. You can pour on some soy/almond/rice milk if you like your grains wet, or just eat as is. You can sweeten your grains with small amounts of either honey or agave—but don't overdo it.

Sprouted bread (not made with flour), such as manna bread, is another good breakfast choice. It's great lightly toasted with any of the allowable spreads, including Tofutti cream cheese, hummus, or nut butters (other than peanut butter).

**If you eat grains for breakfast, consider this your intake of grains for the day and do not have them be part of either of the two remaining meals.**

Some people thrive on protein in the morning. Hemp seed powder, derived from seeds from the hemp plant, is a great source of protein. (Although it's a distant relative of the marijuana plant, it doesn't have any of its mind-altering side effects.) The hemp plant itself has numerous industrial uses—it's even made into cloth. Recently, hemp seeds have been touted as an alternative to milk and soy protein. A hemp protein shake is a great way to start the day easily. It also makes taking your morning supplements easy when you have a thick beverage. If you like going this route, mix the hemp powder with different milk-alternative products. Also, to add a little more substance to the drink, soak a handful of almonds overnight in a covered cup. You will notice that the water fattens them up and makes the skins easy to remove. Wipe off the skins and throw the almonds in the blender with the rest of the drink. You can add extra nutrients and bulk with creatine powder (see page 218).

In sum, any of the allowable protein sources is fair game. Sometimes Dr. Monti will have a leftover piece of salmon for breakfast, which is just fine. Occasionally have eggs if you like (no more than twice per week). Just don't have grains as well.

We also recommend a plant-based protein product called the Ultimate Meal. It's great for those who like to get a little green food in the morning. It is a nutritionally power-packed meal mix, all plant based, that is blended with some fruit and water or soy/rice/almond milk. A few people find it a little bitter, but some of our patients feel that nothing gets them off to a better start.

Some people just don't like the idea of having a full breakfast and prefer to have something light to start off with, followed later by a midmorning snack. That is fine. You can have smaller portions of any of the above, or you can have one of the healthful snacks described below. Do start with something, though. Your body needs fuel in the morning.

Take note of how you feel after eating certain foods. We have had patients discover gluten sensitivities and food allergies simply by paying attention to how their bodies reacted after they ate certain foods. Their "gut feelings" were later confirmed by medical tests.

## Healthful Snacks

- Fruit or soy yogurt.
- Raw vegetables (cucumbers, celery sticks, radishes, etc.) eaten alone or with a dip such as hummus or guacamole. Almond butter, pesto (see recipe), or Tofutti cream cheese (with no dairy) is also good on crackers and vegetables.
- Avoid eating fruits and vegetables together; it's bad for digestion.
- Nuts (see Dan's Trail Mix on page 145).
- Fresh avocado slices on crackers make a great snack.
- Brown rice cakes, or ultra-whole-grain crackers (especially Ryvita crackers), or try one of our favorite brands, Mary's Gone Crackers, with a hummus dip.
- Hemp protein shake mixed with low-sugar rice, almond, or soy milk.

## Lunch and Dinner

These are your vegetable-based meals. We cannot emphasize this enough. We know this many vegetables will take some getting used to for many of you. Again, the majority of the food on your plate for these meals must be vegetables. If three-quarters of your plate is filled with veggies, then any variety of the other categories can make up the remainder: protein sources and whole grains (just don't combine animal protein with grains).

If you do not have a gastrointestinal disorder, eat some raw veggies at one of these meals. Lunch is often when people like to have raw veggies, preferably in the form of a salad (see Dr. Dan's basic salad recipe below).

At least twice a week, have a sprout-based salad. Your body will love you for it (see Anthony's easy sprout recipe below). At the other meal, have as wide a variety of vegetables as you can—at least two. Make sure you eat cruciferous veggies at least four times a week; for both him and her, the middle-years body needs them. The great thing about veggies is that you can eat as much as you like. We have never seen anyone get fat on spinach.

---

### DIET TIP

People often crave ice cream and cereal late at night. These foods give you a rapid rise in blood sugar, which you need for energy. Night cravings are a sign that you need *sleep*, not food.

---

We're not serious cooks, but here are a few simple vegetarian dishes that we make ourselves.

## DAN'S TRAIL MIX

Dan's Trail Mix makes a terrific healthful snack. We offer two different versions of trail mix: one for men and one for women. The Trail Mix for men contains pumpkin seeds, which are good for prostate health. The Trail Mix for women contains flaxseeds, which have been shown to help relieve menopausal symptoms.

1 pound raw almonds
1 pound raw walnuts
½ pound raw sunflower seeds (optional)
¼ pound organic raisins
Pinch of sea salt to taste

*Men: Add ½ cup pumpkin seeds*
*Women: Add ¼ cup ground flaxseeds*

Put all the ingredients in a large plastic storage container, and shake it. Enjoy a trail mix that is more healthful than any trail mix you would buy.

Some: For those who like spicy food, sprinkle a small amount of cayenne pepper on the mixture.

For a change: Heat oven to 325 degrees. Spread trail mix on a baking sheet. Drizzle Bragg Liquid Aminos (it tastes like soy sauce) over the trail mix. Cook for 10 to 15 minutes until mixture is lightly browned. Remove from oven. The trail mix can be eaten at room temperature.

## DAN'S EASY SALAD
1 bag of organic lettuce greens (baby greens, mache, arugula, etc.)
1 small ripe avocado, diced
½ small onion or 2 shallots, finely chopped
1 plum tomato or 4 cherry tomatoes, diced

Place the salad ingredients in a large salad bowl and toss with Dan's Easy Dressing.

### Dan's Easy Dressing`
Assorted fresh herbs (four parts of chopped parsley to whatever other herbs you like, such as chopped basil or sage)
3 ounces cold-pressed extra virgin olive oil
1 small fresh lemon, squeezed

Place the herbs in a small bowl, and mix in the olive oil. Soak the herbs in the oil for at least 15 minutes. Then hand squeeze the lemon into the mixture, lightly whipping it with a fork.

## ANTHONY'S SIMPLE SPROUT SALAD
This is really simple! No measuring spoons needed. Use at least two kinds of sprouts. Put the sprouts in a large bowl, and add enough cold-pressed extra virgin

olive oil to lightly coat them. Add a tablespoon of Bragg Liquid Aminos, and toss the salad. For extra crunch, crumble in one or two brown rice cakes, and toss the salad again.

## PRESTO PESTO

This is usually made with basil, but you can also use parsley or spinach.

1 bunch basil, parsley, or spinach
½ cup finely chopped pine nuts (you can also use walnuts or pecans)
½ cup olive oil

Place the basil (or parsley or spinach) in a food processor or mini-chopper. Chop up the greens until they are fine. Place them in a bowl, and add the pine nuts and olive oil. Stir well. For an even finer consistency, put the mixture in the food processor or mini-chopper one more time.

*Pesto is great over whole grain pasta, brown rice, or on rice cakes.*

---

### HOW BIG IS A SERVING?

1 cup of cereal flakes = the size of a fist
1 cup of raw fruit or vegetables = the size of a fist
1 medium fruit = the size of a baseball
½ cup of cooked fruit or vegetables = the size of ½ baseball
¼ cup of raisins = the size of 1 large egg

---

# RECOMMENDED FOODS

Create your meals from the foods listed below:

| PROTEINS | LOW-CARBOHYDRATE VEGETABLES | OTHER LOW-CARBOHYDRATE VEGETABLES | HIGHER CARBOHYDRATE (to be eaten sparingly) |
|---|---|---|---|
| Plenty of Legumes/Beans; Small Amounts of Some Animal Protein | Greens | Broccoli | No white potatoes in initial 3 weeks |
| Lentils | Kale | Broccoli Rabe | |
| Turkey | Lettuces | Cauliflower | Carrots |
| Soybeans | Cabbage | Artichoke Hearts | Yams |
| Beef | Collard Greens | Brussels Sprouts | Beets |
| Kidney Beans | Spinach | Onions | Sweet Potatoes |
| Chicken | Swiss Chard | Scallions | Peas |
| Black Beans | Watercress | Radishes | Parsnips |
| Eggs | Chicory | Zucchini | White potatoes |
| Chickpeas | Endive | Cucumber | Winter Squashes— |
| Pinto Beans | Escarole | Rhubarb | Butternut, |
| Adzuki Beans, etc. | Chinese Cabbage | Celery | Buttercup Acorn, |
| Bean Products— | Bok Choy | Turnips | Delicata |
| Tofu | Mustard Greens | Peppers | |
| Tempeh | | Jicama | |
| of Fish | | Eggplant | |
| Moderate Amounts | | Avocado | |
| Sole | | Tomato | |
| Flounder | | Water Chestnuts | |
| Tuna | | Bean Sprouts | |
| Salmon | | Snow Pea Pods | |
| Haddock | | Leeks | |
| Monk | | Shallots | |
| Bass | | Spaghetti Squash | |
| Trout | | Asparagus | |
| Sardines, etc. | | Pumpkin | |
| | | String/ Green Beans | |

| SPROUTS (low carb, in a class of their own) | RECOMMENDED NUTS AND SEEDS | GRAINS BUCKWHEAT (KASHA)MILLET | FRUIT* Best Antioxidant Effect |
|---|---|---|---|
| These should be eaten at least twice a week! | Walnuts*** | Rice (Brown!) | Blueberries |
| | Sunflower Seeds*** | Quinoa | Strawberries |
| Broccoli sprouts | Almonds*** | Barley | Raspberries |
| Alfalfa sprouts | Pumpkin Seeds*** | Oats* | Plums |
| Bean sprouts, | Pecans | Millet | Red Grapes |
| etc. | Sesame Seeds*** | Quinoa | Cherries |
| | Macadamia Nuts | Amaranth | Oranges |
| | Pine Nuts (Pignoli) | Rye | |
| | | | *Other* |
| | | *Gluten-sensitive people should avoid wheat and oats, but buckwheat is okay | Apples |
| | | | Apricots |
| | | | Bananas |
| | | | Cherries |
| | | | Figs |
| | | | Grapes |
| | | | Grapefruit |
| | | | Kiwi |
| | | | Mangoes |
| | | | Melons |
| | | | Peaches |
| | | | Pears |
| | | | Pineapple |
| | | | Prunes |
| | | | No more than 2 fruit servings a day as one of the daily snacks or with breakfast. A serving of fruit-flavored, all natural soy yogurt (make sure that it contains less than 10 grams of sugar) can substitute a fruit. |

## PUTTING IT ALL TOGETHER: SUGGESTED MENU FOR WEEK ONE

You can drink spring or filtered water, herbal tea, or decaffeinated green tea with your meals. And yes, you can start with your day with a cup of REAL coffee if you like. We prefer that you use soy or rice milk rather than real milk or cream. Avoid sugar and artificial sweeteners; you may use a ½ teaspoon of *raw* sugar, if needed.

### Day 1

**Breakfast: 3–5** ounces of whole grain mix with soy or rice milk. To make it easy, we recommend having whole grains for breakfast several times a week.

**Midmorning snack:** Three celery sticks with Tofutti cream cheese; you can prepare this at home and bring it to work

**Lunch:** Caesar salad with grilled chicken or tofu, no croutons, light dressing (or hold the dressing and add a little olive oil and a dash of lemon)

**Midday snack:** Handful of Dan's Trail Mix

**Dinner:** Seared tempeh (4- to 6-ounce portions) with lightly steamed broccoli that is then flash-sautéed with garlic

### Day 2

**Breakfast:** Toasted manna bread with almond butter

**Midmorning snack:** Two brown rice cakes or two Ryvita crackers with almond butter

**Lunch:** Sprout salad; if you're at the office, partially prepare at home in advance by simply putting sprouts in a sealed container (Tupperware is good) and having some olive oil, rice cakes, and Bragg Liquid Aminos at the office (you'll want those things there anyway)

**Midday snack:** Handful of Dan's Trail Mix (or individual components of it)

**Dinner:** Tofu (or tempeh) vegetable stir-fry over ½ cup of brown rice; made with lots of cruciferous veggies

## Day 3
**Breakfast:** Whole grains mix as above
**Midmorning snack:** Rice or soy yogurt, as described above
**Lunch:** Organic baby greens with our simple olive oil and lemon dressing and a small (3- to 4-ounce) can of dolphin-safe tuna or wild salmon for her and a 4- to 6-ounce portion for him
**Midday snack:** Fruit option (organic apple, berries, etc.)
**Dinner:** Lentils (cooked or as a thick soup), roasted Brussels sprouts with shallots, and a small grated root salad (one carrot and one beet, finely grated and then drizzled with olive oil)

## Day 4
**Breakfast:** Ultimate Meal or a hemp protein shake
**Midmorning snack:** Brown rice cakes with almond butter
**Lunch:** Chicken vegetable soup, sprinkled with fresh parsley and sage, with a slice of toasted manna bread
**Midday snack:** Trail mix
**Dinner:** Dan's salad with a 4- to 5-ounce grilled salmon fillet for her and a 6-ounce fillet for him; salmon may be substituted by wild mushrooms sautéed in a touch each of olive oil, red wine, and Bragg Liquid Aminos

## Day 5
**Breakfast:** Ultimate Meal or a hemp protein shake
**Midmorning snack:** Rice cakes or cracker option with pesto (if you don't like pesto, substitute one of the other allowable spreads)
**Lunch:** Spinach omelet

**Midday snack:** Piece of fruit (apple, peach, or plum; avoid bananas)

**Dinner:** Chopped asparagus, lightly steamed, then flash-sautéed in olive oil with shiitake mushrooms and a dash of Bragg Liquid Aminos and a pinch of sea salt; cooked millet and cooked cauliflower mashed together with a sprig of sage and 1 tablespoon of Earth Balance spread

## Day 6

**Breakfast:** Hemp shake blended with six to eight raw almonds (ideally soaked overnight and peeled)

**Midmorning snack:** Fruit option

**Lunch:** Black beans (cooked with diced onion or made into a thick soup), and salad of finely chopped cabbage, fresh lemon juice, and 1 tablespoon of soy mayonnaise

**Midday snack:** Zucchini slices with either hummus or another acceptable spread

**Dinner:** Sprout salad (as big as you like, but limit the rice cakes to two)

## Day 7

**Breakfast:** Hemp shake made as above

**Midmorning snack:** Three celery stalks with Tofutti cream cheese

**Lunch:** Miso soup for two with diced tofu and ½ cup of brown rice (you can have the brown rice on the side or put it right in the soup)

**Midday snack:** Nut butter on either two brown rice cakes or an acceptable cracker equivalent

**Dinner:** Large spinach salad for two, topped with bean sprouts; mix in two diced organic hard-boiled eggs and a diced purple onion; use either a low-fat all-natural dressing or our simple olive oil and lemon dressing (optional: add two slices of soy or rice-based cheese)

# IS HE SABOTAGING YOUR DIET?

**HER STORY**

*"My husband is a great guy, but he's trim, and I'm heavier than I want to be. My husband loves ice cream and insists on keeping a few quarts in the freezer for his midnight snack. He can eat a small bowl, but I'll go through the carton. When I ask him not to bring ice cream into the house, he complains that he shouldn't be deprived because I have to lose weight. Who's right?"*

It's counterproductive for the relationship if one spouse feels deprived because the other spouse is working toward weight reduction and a more healthful lifestyle. Now that we've said that, the fact is that while you're dieting you don't need the added temptation of a freezer filled with ice cream. The best approach is for you to ask your husband for help. Don't tell him not to eat ice cream. Instead, say, "I need your support during this difficult time for me. Can you help me out for a while and enjoy your ice cream outside the house while I'm trying to lose weight?" By using this approach, you're enlisting his support as opposed to restricting his activity.

If your husband is uncooperative, try a different tack. You might consider telling your husband that you want to get to a more healthful weight not just for yourself but also because you want him to have a healthier, beautiful partner. Communicate this message: "I want our next several decades to be as good as the first ones, or even better, so I would appreciate your help. Maybe we could get healthier together."

Check out our Web site from time to time, as we will offer new recipes and monthly updates on nutrition (www.greatlifemakeover.com).

## CHAPTER EIGHT

# EXERCISE MAKEOVER

A good mood, good health, good sex, and a fit body are all connected. Many midlife sex problems can be reversed or even prevented by staying physically active. In addition to keeping you trim and toned, regular exercise can prevent many of the physical ailments that can disrupt sexual function. Studies show that regular physical activity can also keep you healthy in several different ways:

- Improve immune function so that your body can resist disease.
- Help you sleep better so that you feel rested and energized.
- Reduce the risk of breast, prostate, and other cancers.
- Decrease inflammation, a contributing factor to many different diseases.
- Keep your muscles and joints strong so that you stay injury free and pain free.
- Relieve stress and anxiety, both of which can make sex the last thing on your mind.
- Promote good digestion and helps to prevent constipation.
- Improve circulation and increases blood flow, which means better sex, healthier-looking skin, and increased vitality.

We developed our workout plan with exercise physiologist Luke Shechtman, who was voted Philadelphia's best personal trainer by Philadelphia's *City Paper*. We ask our midlife couples to work with Luke because he understands the importance of flexibility, balancing major muscle groups, maximizing function, and strengthening the core (trunk muscles)—all vital for maintaining a strong and supple midlife body. Also, check out our Web site (www.greatlifemakeover.com) for monthly fitness updates and tips.

If you are like many of our midlife couples, going to the gym may not fit your lifestyle and schedule. For you, we recommend the following exercises, which can be done at home and can get you and your partner started on a healthful strength-training routine. The program is designed to be done either with a partner or alone. We suggest that you try to work out at least once a week together. It's a good way to keep each other motivated and maintain intimacy.

We also encourage you to invest in a few inexpensive items for your home fitness program. We have selected items that are easily available at almost any sporting goods store or on the internet. They include an exercise ball, at least three exercise resistance bands, a thick exercise mat, and if possible a set of light weights. A bench is optional if you have the room. The total cost of all the equipment is less than the initiation fee charged at many gyms.

We also we urge you to do some form of cardiovascular exercise at least every other day, for about 30 minutes. It will help burn off some of that excess fat, especially around your waist. A brisk walk with your spouse, in which you actually work up a light sweat, is good cardio exercise. (We said "walk," don't run. Running or jogging is not the best exercise for midlife joints.) If you're a member of a gym, you probably have your choice of good exercise machines. For variety, alternate between the elliptical machine, the exercise bike, and the exercise treadmill. Bring your MP3 player—music makes the time fly by. If you have the space and resources, it's not a bad idea to invest in a cardioexercise machine for your home. Exercise bikes and elliptical machines tend to be joint friendly; people with hip or back problems may find it difficult to use an exercise treadmill. Before investing in an exercise machine, try one out at a gym or a friend's house. Some gyms will give you a free trial period before making you sign up, or allow you to pay by the week. It makes sense for you to use a machine a few times to see how it feels before buying one.

Exercise machines can come with lots of fancy gizmos that can jack up the cost, from built-in heart monitors (which can be useful) to TV monitors, which you may not need if you tend to listen to music while you work out or have a TV at home. You're better off buying a pared-down version of a top-of-the-line brand than a souped-up version of a mediocre brand. Trust us: You'll feel the difference once you start working out on a good machine. A well-constructed machine will feel solid, not flimsy.

Portable fold-up models tend to be less expensive than the larger machines and are good for space-challenged homes. There is one downside: because of their smaller size, they are made for smaller bodies. Check the manufacturer's weight recommendations before buying a portable machine. If you are over 200 pounds or so, you are usually better off buying a nonportable machine.

Many people buy exercise machines and don't use them. They haven't yet made the commitment to fitness. Their loss can be your gain. Before buying a new machine, go online or check out the classified section of your local newspaper to see if anyone is selling a used one at a discount. And then make the machine happy—work it out!

In our Exercise Makeover, you will begin with stretching and then move on to strength training. You will end your workout with two core exercises. The entire program should take about 30 minutes. For best results, try to follow the program about three times a week.

Feel free to do the stretching exercises or the core exercises whenever you have time.

## Stretching

Loss of flexibility is a major problem in midlife and is one of the more overlooked elements of fitness and maintaining a fit body. Flexibility helps keep you limber and prevents injury. That's why we recommend that everyone do some stretching every day. In addition, stretching can help counteract those long hours many of us spend hunched over our computers or BlackBerries.

These stretches will start you off on the path toward better posture and a more comfortable daily life. Women are generally more flexible than men, but both have the same need to do basic stretching.

- Hold all stretches for twenty seconds.
- Repeat each stretch up to three times.
- All stretches can be done alone or with a partner.

## HAMSTRING STRETCH

Your hamstrings are the muscles on the back of your legs that support your thighs and butt. If you sit a lot, they can get very stiff and trigger lower back pain.

**A.**

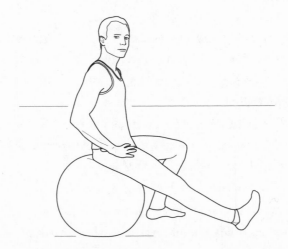

**B.**

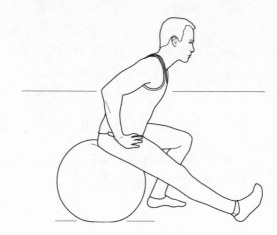

## ALONE

Sit on an exercise ball with your feet firmly planted on the ground. You can also do this exercise sitting on a stable chair or on the side of your bed with your feet on the ground.

Keep your right foot firmly on the ground. Slide your left leg out in front of you, keeping your heel on the ground and your toes in the air.

Slowly bend at your waist until you feel a gradual pull on the back of your thigh. Hold your body straight, with your head up, stomach in, and shoulders back.

Hold the stretch for twenty seconds.

Repeat three times and then switch sides.

## WITH A PARTNER

When you work with a partner, you are doing a "passive" stretch; that is, you allow your partner to move you into a comfortable stretch position. Go for a good stretch, but stop before you experience any pain.

Lie down on your back with your legs extended out in front of you. Your partner is crouched on the floor, facing you.

Your partner holds one of your legs while the other stays extended on the

**A.**

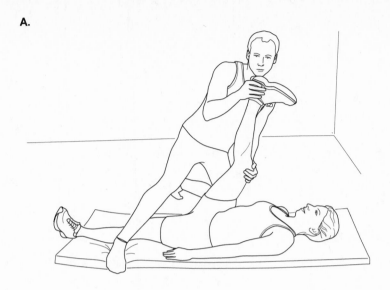

**B.**

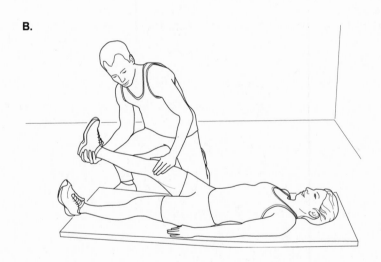

ground. Your partner puts one hand on your heel and one hand on your thigh and gently lifts your leg toward your body until you feel well stretched. (Keep your leg slightly bent at the knee; don't allow your partner to hyperextend it.)

159

This stretch should feel very good, especially if you've been sitting for a long time.

## PECTORAL STRETCH

Your pecs are your chest muscles. Hunching forward makes them stiff and weak. This exercise also helps stretch the arms and shoulders. This exercise is best done with a partner.

### WITH A PARTNER

Sit down on the floor with your legs crossed or bent slightly in front of you and your hands behind your head. Your partner stoops behind you, facing your back. Your partner places his or her knee in between your shoulder blades and slowly pulls back on your elbows until you feel the stretch.

Hold for twenty seconds and release. Repeat three times.

A.

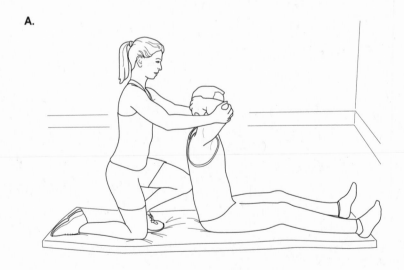

**B.**

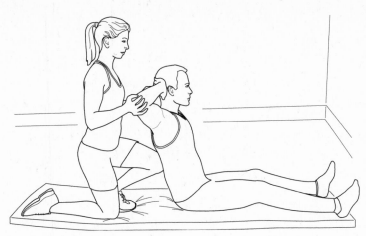

## LATISSIMUS STRETCH

**Equipment Needed: Exercise Ball**

Your lats are your upper back muscles.

**A.**

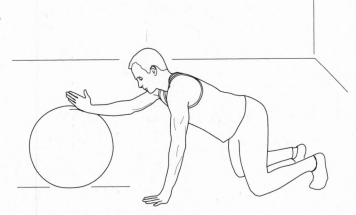

B.

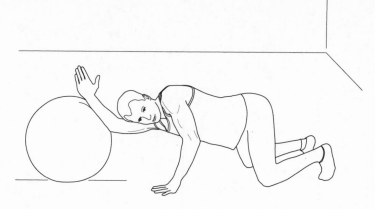

## WITH A PARTNER

Kneel down on your knees behind the ball. Put one of your hands in a karate-chop position on top of the ball, while the other stabilizes you on the floor.

Slowly lower your chest, leaning on the ball, until you feel a stretch in your armpit. The round surface of the ball can be used to move and manipulate the stretch. Your partner should stand in front of the ball to help stabilize it, especially as you are getting used to this stretch.

Hold for twenty seconds. Repeat three times, then switch arms.

# CALF STRETCH

This is the classic stretch. It's good for women who wear high heels and find that their legs hurt the next day! But it's important for men, too.

## ALONE

Stand at the bottom of a staircase and hold on to the railing with one hand.

Place the balls of your feet on the step, leaving your heels off the step.

Slowly lower your heels until you feel a tight stretch behind your shin.

A.　　　　　　　　　　　　B.

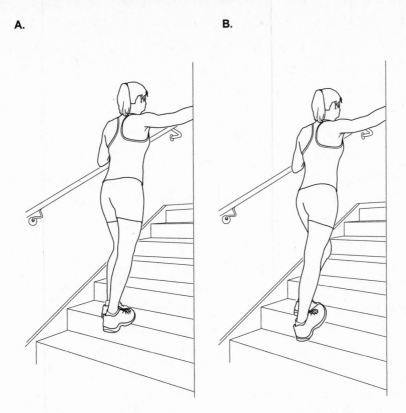

## WITH A PARTNER

Lie flat on your back with your partner sitting at your feet. Your partner takes your foot in his or her hand and presses the heel up against the chest until you feel a mild stretch.

Hold the stretch for twenty seconds. Repeat three times and then switch to the other foot.

## Strength Training

In the past, women have been viewed as the physically weaker sex, and it was the men who were encouraged to lift weights and build muscle mass. Women were relegated to the aerobics area of the gym. Today we know that this concept is incorrect. Men and women have the same musculoskeletal need for strength training. It helps maintain muscle mass and increase bone density, which are especially important for postmenopausal women. Strength training also helps decrease body fat, increase lean muscle, and maintain correct posture.

If you're someone who likes to work out at the gym or with a personal fitness coach, great. Now's the time to reaffirm your commitment to exercise. But you can certainly do any of these exercises at home or on the road if you travel a lot.

Once you become familiar with how to use resistance bands, you can use them instead of weights to get a great workout just about anywhere. But you have to use them safely. Be sure to attach them securely to a **stable** object, such as doorknobs, bed frames, and radiators. As an added bonus, they are easily transportable and take up little room in your travel bag. By standing in the middle of the band and holding one end in each hand, you can curl, overhead press, triceps extend, and do multiple exercises for the shoulders and back. The tauter the band, the harder the resistance. If you wrap the middle of the band around a doorknob, you can lunge, chest press, row, and even rotate laterally to work on those pesky love handles.

Men and women tend to store fat in different places of the body. Men often put on weight around the midsection, while women tend to gain in the hips, legs, and buttocks area. Even though we all should be doing our best to get a full-body workout by emphasizing all major muscle groups, it's okay to focus a little more on those areas that tend to bother you the most.

All exercises should be done with slow, controlled movements, with little to no pause between reps and, most important, with good form. Allow thirty to sixty seconds between sets. When you do the exercises this way, there will be a significant cardio component to the workout as well.

Do three sets of ten to twelve reps for each exercise. The last three reps should be difficult.

For each repetition, count one, two on the exertion and one, two, three on the release.

# SQUATS

Good form is essential for squats to keep you from putting too much pressure on your back or your knees.

Stand straight with your feet hip-width apart and with your hands on your hips. Be sure that your shoulders are not hunched forward, your head is erect, and your chin is up.

Roll your hips forward so that your butt slides back. Hold your stomach in tight.

Slowly lower your body down, but don't allow your knees to extend beyond 90 degrees. *Make sure that your knees don't extend over your toes.* Lift yourself back up to the starting position. Be sure to maintain your posture.

## VARIATION

A good variation for women is the plié squat. It's performed the same way as the standard squat, but instead of keeping your feet straight, you point your toes outward. This gives your hips, thighs, and glutes a better workout.

**A.**    **B.**

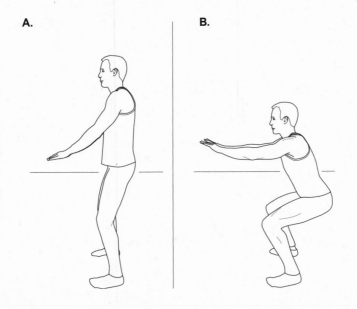

# SHOULDERS

### Lateral Arm Raise

This exercise gives your shoulders a workout. It is good for toning and shaping.

Stand up tall with your feet shoulder-width apart and your knees slightly bent.

**A.**

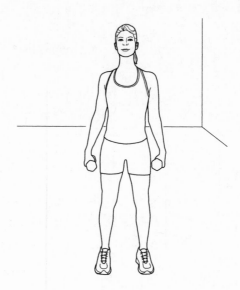

**B.**

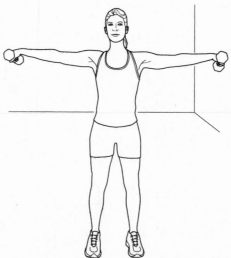

Grab a *light* weight (between 3 and 5 pounds) in either hand. Place your arms at your sides with your palms down.

Slightly bend your elbows, and slowly lift your arms out sideways to bring the weights to chest level. Lower the weights back to starting position.

Do three sets of ten to twelve reps.

## Front Raise

Stand up tall with your feet shoulder-width apart and your knees slightly bent.

Grab a *light* weight (between 3 and 5 pounds) in either hand as if you are holding a hammer. Place your arms at your sides.

Slightly bend your elbows, and slowly raise the weights to chest level.

Do three sets of ten to twelve reps.

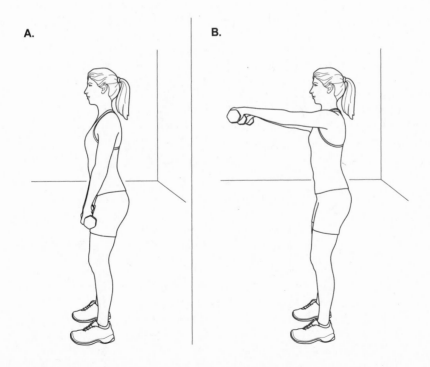

A.

B.

# BACK

### Bent-Over Row

A bent-over row is a back exercise usually performed with a weight. You work one side of your body, and then switch and do the other. Ideally, this exercise is performed on a bench, but it can also be done on the side of a bed.

**A.**

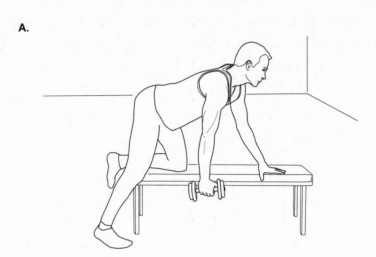

**B.**

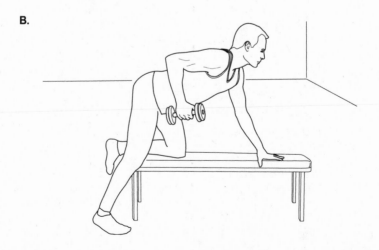

Place your left leg and left hand on the bench while keeping your right foot firmly planted on the ground. Keep your back as flat as possible.

Pick up a weight with your right hand. Keeping your arm close to your body, bring the weight up to your chest. Your elbow should be pointing to the ceiling, and your head should be erect. Don't let your back curve in.

Release slowly back to starting position. Do three sets of ten to twelve reps.

Switch sides and repeat exercise.

# CHEST

### Bench Press

Lie on your back with your weights in your hands, placed beside your chest. Keep your palms facing down.

Slowly straighten your arms until the weights are at your chest.

Lower to starting position. Do three sets of ten to twelve reps.

**A.**

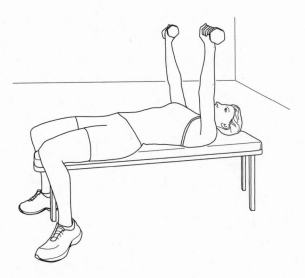

**B.**

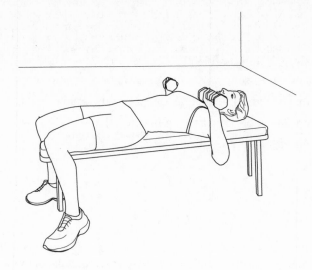

## BICEPS

### Curls

These exercises can be done with any of numerous pieces of equipment. While not as functional a muscle group as some of the others, the biceps and forearms are easy to

**A.**          **B.**

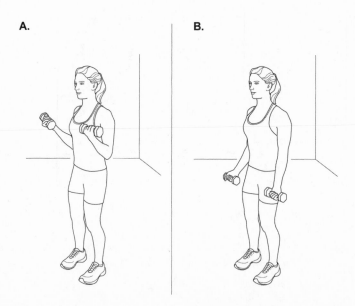

tone, they look attractive in both men and women when toned, and they are good for self-esteem, especially when you are wearing short-sleeved shirts or sleeveless dresses.

Stand with your feet shoulder-width apart, and pick up a weight in either hand. Place your arms at your sides, palms up, with your elbows close to your sides.

Curl your arms until your elbows bend past 90 degrees.

Lower to starting position. Do three sets of ten to twelve reps.

## TRICEPS

### Modified Push-up

Get on your hands and knees, on a mat or heavy towel. Your palms are flat on the ground, and your elbows are at your sides. Your neck is straight, and you are holding your stomach in tight.

While keeping your neck straight, lower yourself down until your head is about 6 inches from the floor.

Then push up until your back is flat. Keep holding your stomach in tight to avoid letting your back sink in.

Return to starting position.

Do three sets of ten to twelve reps.

**A.**

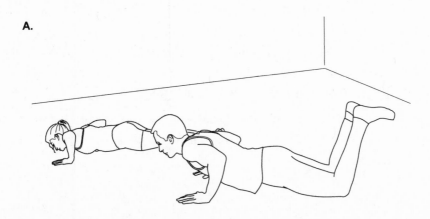

B.

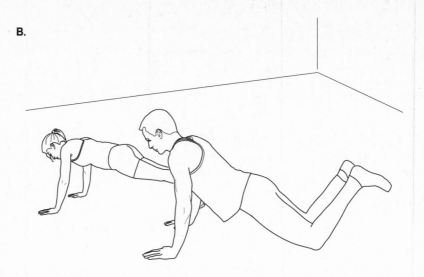

## HIPS AND GLUTES

### Lateral Leg Raise

Stand with your feet shoulder-width apart, your legs slightly bent at the knees.

Find something about waist level (such as a sturdy table or desk) to grab on to with one arm to help keep you stable. Also, hold your stomach in tight to keep from wobbling. Your stomach, not your arm, should be doing the work to hold you up.

Slowly raise your leg to the side until it is nearly straight, or as far as you can go.

Lower your leg to starting position.

Do three sets of ten to twelve reps. Then switch legs and repeat the exercise.

This is a wonderful exercise for women who want to tone the outer hip and gluteal area. If you want to challenge yourself, add resistance by attaching a resistance band or adding a leg weight.

A.

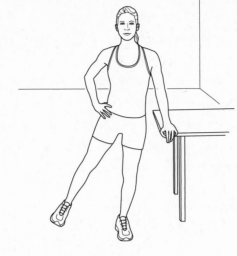

B.

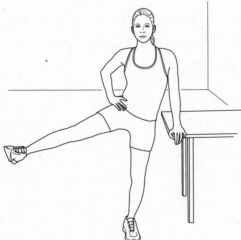

## Core Exercises

For years we have been told to train the body one or two muscle groups at a time. This was known as the body-building workout, and if you wanted to get "big," that was the way to do it. This method is somewhat effective, but because of the specificity of the training, it leaves the body vulnerable to everyday movements. Today we take a more functional approach with our training by emphasizing the core. The core consists of the muscles that run the entire length of the torso and stabilize the spine and pelvis. These muscles provide a solid base for movement in the extremities. Including core exercises in your routine will make it easier to stand upright and to move on two feet. They will also help you control your body and control weight shift when the body moves in different directions. Here are a couple of core exercises to start with.

## CORE ROTATION

Stand with your feet shoulder-width apart and your legs slightly bent at the knees. Hold your stomach in tight, and keep your feet stable.

**A.**

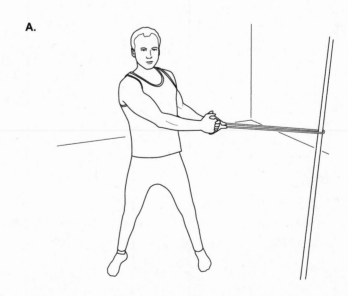

**B.**

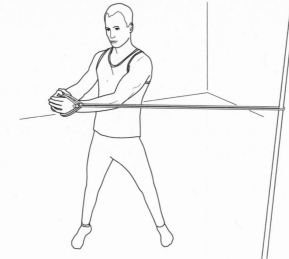

Grab one end of the exercise band in each hand. Hold your arms out in front of you at chest level. Keep the band straight and taut.

Rotate the band across your body as you twist to one side.

Repeat this movement until your torso is tired; then turn around and repeat the exercise.

This exercise can also be done with a partner, using the resistance band. Each individual grips one handle of the band, and the two then move in opposite directions, creating resistance.

Do three sets of ten to twelve reps.

## FRONT STABILIZATION

Lie flat on a mat facedown, with your knees bent and your arms bent so that your elbows are on the mat. Suck your stomach in, and slowly lift your torso about 8 inches off the ground.

**A.**

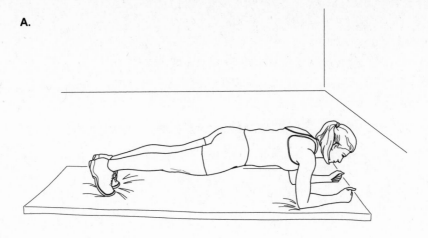

**B.**

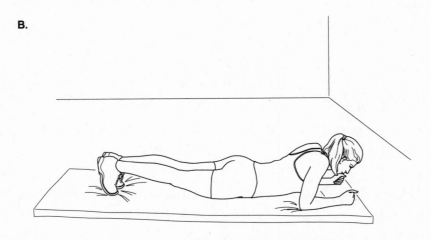

Control your breathing as you continue to hold that position.

Lower yourself back to your starting position.

Do three sets of ten to twelve reps.

And yes, this is hard to do!

## CHAPTER NINE

# HORMONE MAKEOVER

The three hot-button issues of midlife—sexual problems, weight, and mood—are all affected by hormonal changes that occur during these years for both men and women. Diet, exercise, and stress reduction can help maintain a youthful body and a sharp mind. For some people, losing weight, starting a regular exercise program, and living a more balanced life are all it takes to look and feel better. In effect, they are rebalancing their hormones through lifestyle changes and using the supplements we recommend on page 211. If you are one of these lucky people, then you don't need to consider doing anything more.

For others, lifestyle interventions aren't enough. They may find that the midlife decline in hormone production is accelerating the aging process and sending them on a downward spiral that interferes with both their health and their quality of life. When more help is needed, there's another option—hormone replacement therapy (HRT) using what are called bioequivalent hormones (BHRT). Bioequivalent hormones are sometimes referred to as natural hormones to distinguish them from the synthetic non-bioequivalent hormones used in standard HRT.

Some of you may be thinking, "Aren't hormones dangerous?" or "My doctor took me off hormones because she said they cause cancer." These are legitimate concerns, which we will address in this chapter. There is a tremendous confusion and controversy surrounding the use of any types of hormones, bioequivalent and NON-bioequivalent. As many of you know, HRT has been linked to an increased risk of breast cancer, but only after it was prescribed to millions of women for several decades. The medical community's complete reversal on HRT has made many women angry at their doctors and wary of all hormone therapy.

Many women, however, have weighed the risks and decided to take hormones anyway. A vocal group of doctors and lay people have been touting the safety of bioequivalent hormones, claiming that unlike synthetic hormones, they don't cause cancer. Their assertions have elicited a strong and negative response from the mainstream medical community—including some leading cancer specialists—who contend that there is no difference between bioequivalent and synthetic hormones, and who caution against using any form of HRT.

Testosterone replacement is controversial, too, but for different reasons. Today, millions of men are using testosterone replacement to treat low testosterone levels. Nearly all the prescriptions written for testosterone today are for a bioequivalent form of the hormone, which many people think is better. Still, some physicians question whether testosterone replacement is safe, and a sizable minority don't believe that midlife men need to replenish sinking testosterone levels.

The debate over hormones has become very emotional. This is unfortunate. Before people can make an appropriate decision about whether or not to use BHRT, they need to arm themselves with the facts. The purpose of this chapter is to provide a comprehensive look at the available options for men and women who are considering BHRT.

Before we get started, we'd like to state our position on hormones so you know where we stand. First, we believe that BHRT is not the same as HRT and that consumers (and some doctors) need to understand the difference. If you do decide to take hormones, we urge you to strongly consider using bioequivalent hormones. Although they may have been more difficult to get in the past, BHRT products are widely prescribed and available in most pharmacies today. You can also obtain them through a compounding pharmacy that produces customized hormone preparations based on your doctor's prescription. By the time you've finished reading this chapter, you'll understand why we feel so strongly about using BHRT.

Second—and this is a very important point—although we believe that if BHRT is done appropriately, it can benefit many men and women, it is not for everyone. The decision to take BHRT depends on your medical history, your overall health, and your goals. Many questions about BHRT for men and women have not been answered, and to date, no large-scale studies have investigated its safety. Nevertheless, we believe that it's possible for men and women to make an intelligent decision based on available information.

In the first part of this chapter, we review BHRT options for women. In the second part, we discuss testosterone replacement for men. We urge men and women to read both sections because we cover different aspects of hormone replacement in each one. Furthermore, reading both sections will help you better understand what your partner is going through, and you may be able to help him or her make a better decision.

## HER HORMONE MAKEOVER

There are two schools of thought about hormone replacement for women. One group favors using hormone replacement solely for treating menopausal symptoms and nothing more. They believe that if a woman has such severe menopausal symptoms that nothing else can help, she should take hormones in the *lowest dose for the shortest amount of time*. Many mainstream practitioners today fall into this category. They don't differentiate between using standard synthetic hormones (standard HRT) or bioequivalent hormones unless the patient expresses a preference.

The other group favors using hormone replacement strategically to help keep people stronger and healthier as they approach their later decades. They believe that hormones should be taken at physiologic doses (brought back up to their youthful levels) to prevent age-related damage and to maintain maximum mental and physical function. We tend to fall somewhere in between, and whichever approach we use, we follow some very clear guidelines and safety precautions.

In our practice, we typically see women who seek us out specifically because of our hormone rebalancing program. These women are already convinced that they want BHRT to prevent—and reverse—the age-related changes they see happening to them as they reach menopause. They are part of a growing number of women and men who have made a conscious choice that they want to grow older in youthful, vital bodies. They don't want to get flabby, lose inches of height to osteoporosis, or have their sex lives disrupted by vaginal thinning and dryness. They believe that BHRT will help keep them young for as long as possible. We feel that along with a healthful lifestyle, BHRT can be useful in helping them achieve their goals.

We also treat women who view BHRT as a short-term solution to help them cope with severe menopausal symptoms. These women may be worried about the long-term effects of hormones, but they are so unhappy about their hot flashes, insomnia, and mood swings that they're willing to take hormones for a short time. We respect their point of view, and we work with them also.

We also see women who have previously taken synthetic hormones and felt good while taking them but discontinued them because of the negative reports. For the first time in years, many of these women are now confronted with menopausal symptoms. They are seeking an effective way to enjoy the benefits of hormone replacement while minimize the health risks of synthetic hormones.

BHRT can help a woman stave off some age-related changes that occur after menopause. Most of the sexual problems discussed in Chapter 1, from vaginal dryness and thinning, to difficulties achieving orgasm, to low libido, can be treated effectively with BHRT.

We tailor our program to suit each woman's needs and goals. There are risks involved in any drug or medical intervention, and these risks vary from woman to woman. Before we prescribe BHRT to a woman, we take a careful patient history and perform the appropriate medical tests to make sure that she doesn't have any underlying medical problem that could be aggravated by taking hormones.

## HRT: A BRIEF HISTORY

At its inception about five decades ago, HRT was touted as a "cure" for menopause. Estrogen replacement was first given to women in the 1950s who had undergone hysterectomies and were thrown into early menopause. It relieved their symptoms so well that doctors began prescribing estrogen to women who had reached menopause naturally but were hard hit by hot flashes and other symptoms. Many women liked how they felt on estrogen, and they wanted to stay on it indefinitely.

Estrogen users enjoyed some definite benefits, including the positive sexual side effects that prevented the normal changes in vaginal tone and difficulties with orgasm. Women noticed that their skin stayed more supple on estrogen, their breasts stayed firmer, and they looked and felt better than their friends who were not taking estrogen.

In 1968, Robert Wilson, M.D., wrote a bestselling book, *Feminine Forever,* which touted estrogen replacement as a antiaging breakthrough that enabled women to remain "fully feminine—physically and emotionally—for as long as they live." The book would be considered very sexist today because it suggested that once a woman went through menopause, she was by definition sexually undesirable. Nevertheless, *Feminine Forever* had a very seductive message: it told women that there was a simple way to stay sexy and young. It hit a nerve and became a major best seller. What wasn't known at the time was that Dr. Wilson was an unofficial spokesperson for Wyeth-Ayerst, the manufacturers of Premarin (short for pregnant-mare urine), a synthetic estrogen that blended more than ten different types of estrogens found in the urine of pregnant mares. Sales for Premarin skyrocketed after the publication of the book, and HRT became mainstream.

The estrogen bubble was burst in 1972, when a study of women taking estrogen alone revealed higher rates of endometrial or uterine cancer. Progestin, a synthetic progesterone, was added to estrogen therapy to prevent the buildup of the uterine lining in a manner similar to the role progesterone plays in the menstrual cycle. The addition of progestin eliminated the increased risk for uterine cancer but may have caused other problems down the road.

Researchers—some funded by pharmaceutical companies— became interested in studying the effects of HRT on women's health. Several small-scale studies found that HRT not only was effective at eliminating menopausal symptoms but possibly could offer significant health benefits in terms of preventing diseases such as osteoporosis, heart disease, Alzheimer's disease, and colon cancer. The fact that HRT was supposed to prevent many of the so-called diseases of aging was heralded as great news, particularly since tens of millions of American baby-boomer women were heading toward menopause. Medical journals ran editorials chastising doctors for not prescribing HRT for all menopausal women.

## MILLIONS OF WOMEN ON HRT

By the turn of the twenty-first century, more than 10 million postmenopausal American women were taking synthetic estrogen, usually Premarin. Most women were taking Premarin plus progestin, a synthetic progesterone, marketed in a combination pill called PREMPRO.

Women's health advocates began to question whether it was wise for so many women to be using HRT on the basis of so few studies. In response to critics, the National Institutes of Health (NIH) launched the first large-scale study of HRT— the Women's Health Initiative (WHI) study—in the mid-1990s. Researchers observed 16,000 postmenopausal women of median age in their early 60s who were without symptoms and who (1) still had a uterus and (2) were taking a combination synthetic estrogen-progestin drug or a placebo. Much to their chagrin, after five years, researchers found that there was a significant increase in heart disease, blood clots, stroke, and invasive breast cancer among women taking the hormones versus those taking the placebo.

In 2002, researchers became so convinced that HRT was putting women's lives at risk that they called off the study three years early. A year later, further review of the data revealed an increased risk of breast cancer and cardiovascular events (such as heart attack and stroke) in women taking HRT. Despite earlier hopes that HRT would help prevent colorectal cancer, it appeared to have no impact either positively or negatively.

The Heart/Estrogen Progestin Replacement Study (HERS Study), launched in 1993, investigated estrogen and heart disease. By 1998, the HERS study reported that women taking HRT did not have lower rates of heart disease than did placebo takers. The study raised a red flag: women who had had previous heart disease were at an increased risk of having a second cardiovascular event if they took HRT. By 2002, the HERS trial found absolutely no advantage to taking HRT in terms of cardiovascular health.

The news went from bad to worse. In 2003, the WHI found that PREMPRO doubled the risk of dementia in women over 65. In 2004, the WHI found that the estrogen-only group had an increased risk of stroke, and those women were taken off Premarin for good.

HRT wasn't all bad. It decreased the risk for hip fractures and other fractures, and it did a good job in preventing menopausal symptoms such as hot flashes, vaginal thinning, and mood swings for millions of women.

## Sorting Through the Science

The WHI and HERS trials had a chilling effect on HRT, and practically overnight, millions of women were abruptly taken off hormones. Many women were led to believe that their only option was to risk disease or suffer through menopausal symptoms.

After the initial news coverage of the WHI and HERS trials, other facts emerged that were not reported by the media but were very important in shedding light on HRT. Subanalyses of the WHI study and several subsequent articles showed that *estrogen alone does not appear to increase breast cancer.* In fact, the real culprit appears to be synthetic progestins.

In 2004, at the same time researchers reported on the higher rate of blood clots among the estrogen-only users, they also found that women taking estrogen alone did not have a higher risk of breast cancer, heart disease, or blood clots in the lungs. Further analysis of the data showed that women who had the highest rates of breast cancer were taking combination therapy that included progestin. However, other studies have shown that *natural progesterone* may have a *protective effect* against breast cancer.

There are yet more twists and turns in the estrogen story. An April 2008 study published in the *Journal of the National Cancer Institute* reported that further analysis of the WHI data showed that women taking Premarin alone had "a statistically significant increased risk of benign proliferative breast disease" (breast lumps), a condition associated with an increased risk of breast cancer. So, although these women did not initially have a higher rate of breast cancer, they could be at greater risk down the road.

The bottom line: Estrogen alone—even the chemically produced, estrogen-like commercial Premarin—did not appear to increase the risk of breast cancer, at least over the span of the study. The recently reported increased incidence of benign breast lumps in women taking Premarin is an ominous warning sign that estrogen alone—or this artificial form of estrogen-like chemicals—may, over time, cause an increase in cancer. Estrogen-like compounds, if taken orally, however, do increase the risk of blood clots. Progestin—fake progesterone—increases the risk of breast cancer.

Taken together, synthetic estrogen and progestin increase the risk of breast cancer, heart disease, and dementia.

Frankly, we were not surprised by the results of the WHI study. We believe that synthetic hormones, *particularly progestins*, are dangerous and are not comparable to bio-identical hormones. They are artificial imposters that may at times partly behave like the original hormones, but are not comparable to the real thing. Some of the common synthetic hormones are much more potent than the hormones used in BHRT, and your body knows the difference.

## THE BHRT DIFFERENCE

We do not prescribe "synthetic," or, more correctly, "NON-bioequivalent" hormones because we don't think they are the best option. We prescribe bioequivalent hormones. There is a big difference between bioequivalent and NON-bioequivalent, but there are also some similarities.

Critics of BHRT often claim that when these substances are obtained from a compounding pharmacy, they are less regulated and may come from questionable sources. This is usually not true. It may surprise you to learn that most hormones, whether they are bioequivalent or NON-bioequivalent, are made from two plant sources—wild yam or soy-based products—which are also used by major drug companies. In other words, the raw material used to make bioequivalent hormones is the same stuff used by the manufacturers who make non-bioequivalent hormones. The manufacturers of the raw materials sell the same bioequivalent hormone preparations to pharmaceutical companies that make proprietary hormone products and to compounding pharmacies that produce customized preparations in the form of gels, creams, or pellets of the unchanged bioequivalent hormones.

So the real difference is that pharmaceutical companies often manipulate the chemical structure of a hormone and alter it, making it something other than the precise formula of the hormones in your body. It is close enough to create biological activity in your body similar to the original hormone, but it is many times more potent. That's why we call this a non-bioequivalent hormone.

In the case of a bioequivalent hormone, as above, the raw plant material is converted into a hormone that is *chemically identical* to the hormone found in the human body—a bioequivalent hormone. Please note that it is not an actual human hormone but an identical chemical copy that behaves like the real thing. As described above, it is then sold to a pharmaceutical company, or a compounding pharmacist, a licensed pharmacist who uses it to fill prescriptions written by doctors for individual patients.

Why make non-bioequivalent hormones? Why tinker with Mother Nature?

The answer has more to do with profits than with patient care. Hormones are natural substances and therefore cannot be patented. In this case, you are actually penalized for making a substance that is identical to nature. In order to obtain a patent for a hormone, you have to deviate from the original design. The end product may have hormone-like tendencies—it may behave like a hormone and have many of the same effects as a hormone—but it is no longer identical to the hormone in the human body. And we believe, with support like the WHI study, that these synthetic hormones are far riskier and have a much greater potential for harm than bioequivalent hormones. Given what we know about biochemistry, combined with our clinical experience, we are concerned that synthetic hormones may be more likely to produce harmful byproducts that can (1) promote blood clots and (2) stimulate the growth of hormone-sensitive cancers.

Why do pharmaceutical companies also market some bioequivalent hormones? They do so because they can patent the delivery system, such as a patch or a gel.

We prescribe bioequivalent hormones sold by pharmaceutical companies (e.g., AndroGel for men), and we also use compounding pharmacies for certain BHRT products, such as pellets.

Another distinction is that bioequivalent hormones obtained from a compounding pharmacy can be specifically dosed by the physician, allowing for more precision in meeting the needs of particular patients, while a pharmaceutical company's products, whether synthetic or bioequivalent, are predosed and prepackaged, which makes dosing far less precise. This is sometimes an issue and other times not a big deal. It depends on the patient and how and why we are using the hormones.

Are bioequivalent hormones safe? A few small studies suggest that BHRT is safe, but in the absence of a large-scale long-term study, there is no definitive answer. We can't make a blanket statement that bioequivalent hormones are completely safe for all women. That would be irresponsible. There are some women for whom the risk of taking hormones may outweigh any benefits. Women at very high risk for breast cancer may fall into this category. We believe strongly that each case should be taken individually.

## THE PHYSICAL EXAM FOR WOMEN

Before we prescribe BHRT to a woman, we first do a complete history and physical examination to (1) make sure that she is in good health, (2) determine if she is a good candidate for hormones, and (3) tailor a prescription to meet her needs.

We ask every patient to fill out a detailed questionnaire about her health and lifestyle. This gives our patients an opportunity to express their needs and desires and also provides us with a detailed history. When we meet the patient, we have an excellent platform from which to start making medical decisions.

What tests should women have, and when should they have them? Below, we offer our general guidelines for medical tests based on gender and age. Your physician may recommend additional tests or more rigorous follow-up based on your family or medical history.

## PREVENTIVE HEALTH EXAM

At age 20, all women should have a complete fasting lipid profile performed every five years. If you have a lipid imbalance, your doctor may require this test to be done more frequently.

Starting at age 40, all women should have a comprehensive physical examination, including a detailed family medical history, all basic lab tests, a blood pressure check, and a review of potential risk factors.

Height and weight should be taken at each visit and carefully monitored. The basic preventive health exam should be repeated at least every three years until age 50.

Starting at age 50, the preventive health exam should be done every two years. By age 65, it should be done annually.

After age 65, vision and hearing should be checked annually as part of the exam.

### Diabetes Screen

All adults with high blood pressure or dyslipidemia (bad blood fats) should be given a fasting plasma glucose test to screen for diabetes.

### Colon Cancer Screen

Starting at age 50, all women should have a colonoscopy every three to five years. After age 80, this test should be done at the discretion of the patient and the doctor.

### Breast Cancer Screening

Starting at age 40, all women should do a breast self-exam monthly and report any changes to their physicians.

Starting at age 40, all women should have a mammogram every one or two years. An annual mammogram is especially important if you are using either BHRT or HRT. Many breast tumors are estrogen sensitive, which means that some forms of estrogen can stimulate their growth.

Women with existing breast cancer should not take BHRT, with very rare exceptions. (Some experts believe that short-term BHRT may be appropriate for carefully selected breast cancer survivors who have severe symptoms of estrogen deficiency.)

After age 70, mammograms should be performed at the physician's discretion.

### Cervical Cancer Screening

Starting at age 21, or within three years of the onset of sexual activity, every woman should have a Pap smear every three years. Pap smears are not necessary after age 70 if three or more Pap smears in a row have been normal, there have been no abnormal Pap smears within the past ten years, and the woman is not at high risk.

### Osteoporosis Screening

Starting at age 50, all women should have a baseline DEXA bone density test. If the woman is not at high risk for osteoporosis, the test can be repeated every few years at her physician's discretion. If she is at high risk for fractures, the test should be repeated more often. At age 65, ALL women should have routine DEXA tests (every year or so) as part of their physical exam.

### Baseline Bone Scan

The first five years of menopause are marked by a rapid loss of bone mass. A baseline bone scan (DEXA scan) can help a woman and her doctor track how much bone she is losing, to determine if BHRT should be considered to prevent osteoporosis.

### Transvaginal Ultrasound

If a woman has a history of fibroid tumors or unusual menstrual symptoms, we may also perform a vaginal ultrasound to examine the reproductive organs, such as the endometrium (uterine lining) and ovaries. Although many insurance companies don't pay for routine transvaginal ultrasound, this quick and painless test is a good way to detect abnormalities and possibly even cancer in its early and most treatable stages.

### Check Levels of Key Hormones

If a woman complains of typical menopausal symptoms, we order a hormone panel to check her levels of key hormones. This is the most accurate way to assess whether she is truly menopausal, and determine which hormones she may need to replace.

## FOLLICLE-STIMULATING HORMONE (FSH)

In the menstrual cycle, FSH tells the ovaries to produce estrogen. As estrogen production begins to wane during perimenopause and menopause, FSH levels rise in an attempt to rev up estrogen production by the ovaries. Rising FSH levels produce some of the most unpleasant symptoms of menopause.

## ESTRADIOL

There are three forms of estrogen in the female body: estradiol, estrone, and estriol. Estradiol is the most important female hormone in that it regulates the menstrual cycle, is crucial for bone density, and is important for mood, sex drive, brain function, and even skin elasticity. The loss of estradiol is what triggers most of the symptoms we associate with menopause. Not surprisingly, estradiol is the primary estrogen used in BHRT. When women have symptoms such as vaginal dryness, night sweats, hot flashes, and moodiness, a consistently high FSH level combined with a low estradiol level strongly points to menopause-induced hormone deficiency.

## ESTRONE

Estrone is the most problematic of the estrogens because it is potentially carcinogenic. After menopause, estrone levels actually rise. Both estradiol and estrone have the same potential breakdown products.

## TESTOSTERONE (TOTAL AND FREE)

Although testosterone is essential for a woman's health and well-being, her body makes very little of this hormone. Even a minor dip in testosterone can have adverse affects in terms of sex drive, energy, mood, and bone mass. There are several ways to evaluate testosterone: there's total testosterone, free testosterone, and a protein called sex-hormone-binding globulin, or SHBG. In both men and women, most testosterone is bound to SHBG and albumin and is released into the bloodstream as needed. Only a very small amount (2%) of total testosterone in the body is free testosterone—that is, unbound and available for use by our cells and tissues. As we age, the amount of testosterone on SHBG increases, leaving less testosterone for our use. If you measure only total testosterone, you may get a false impression of how much testosterone is actually available. It's possible for a woman to have a normal total testosterone level but still be deficient in free testosterone. There is some controversy as to the accuracy of the free testosterone measurement. We try to obtain as complete a picture of clinical and lab data as possible to guide us in working with each particular patient.

## PROGESTERONE

Synthetic progestins were added to HRT as an afterthought to prevent endometrial cancer. Natural progesterone, which is produced by the ovaries, the adrenal glands, and the brain, plays an important role in maintaining mood and brain function. When levels of progesterone sink too low, a woman may experience sleep problems, anxiety, and irritability. If a woman is taking estrogen and she still has her uterus, she must also take progesterone. Progesterone levels may drop faster and more steeply than estrogen, and some women who are still menstruating may take natural progesterone before they need estrogen replacement.

## SEX-HORMONE-BINDING GLOBULIN (SHBG)

Sex steroids are carried in the blood on carrier proteins. Less than 2% circulate in the unbound form, and these hormones are in a form that can actually go into the cells and tissues where they are needed. SHBG is such a carrier protein, with an important role in regulating the amount of unbound steroids in the blood. It binds strongly with testosterone and dihydrotestosterone (DHT), a testosterone metabolite, and less strongly with estradiol. *It reduces the activity of the sex hormones.* High levels of SHBG suggest that there is not enough of one or more steroids in their free form.

## THYROID-STIMULATING HORMONE (TSH)

Thyroid hormone deficiency can be common among midlife women and often goes undetected because it produces many of the same symptoms associated with menopause, including fatigue, irritability, menstrual problems, dry skin, and memory problems. TSH will be elevated if there is not enough thyroid hormone in circulation. If thyroid levels are low, thyroid hormone can be taken to bring levels back to normal.

## Check Levels of Estrogen Metabolites

Whether estrogen is taken as HRT or is made by the body, it is broken down or metabolized into byproducts called metabolites. Specifically, there are two types of estrogen metabolic groups that can be made by the body: catechol estrogens and methyl estrogens. Catechol estrogens, which often progress to form semiquinones or quinones, seem to be carcinogenic; these estrogens damage DNA and can fuel the growth of estrogen-dependent cancers, including many breast cancers. On the other hand, methylation of estrogens tends to make them benign and may even block the growth of tumors. Although we don't yet know the whole story, we believe that a combination of genetics, dietary factors, and lifestyle factors make some women more prone to make primarily "bad" estrogen (catechol), while others make mostly good estrogen metabolites.

Before we prescribe BHRT, we routinely order a blood test to screen for the ratios of dangerous versus desirable estrogen metabolites. If a woman learns that she makes more of the bad estrogen than the "good" kind, the situation is not hopeless. She doesn't have to sit around and wait for cancer to strike. She can take steps to alter the estrogen pathways from making more bad estrogen to making more good estrogen. Cruciferous vegetables (broccoli, kale, Brussels sprouts, cabbage) in particular contain high amounts of factors that favor the formation of good estrogen metabolites. All women should eat lots of these vegetables, but especially women who produce more bad estrogen metabolites. We also recommend three additional supplements, described on page 220, that have been shown to decrease formation of the toxic estrogens.

After making dietary changes and prescribing the supplements, we do periodic blood tests to check for improvement in the ratios of bad to good estrogen metabolites. Although this is not part of the usual medical workup for women, we believe that it will eventually be standard protocol for the prevention of estrogen-dependent cancers and for HRT in the future. Typically, we see a significant improvement in estrogen metabolite ratios in most, but not all, women.

If we discover that a woman is prone to make high levels of cancer-causing estrogen metabolites, it doesn't mean that she can never take hormones, but we very carefully consider her situation. We first recommend that she make the appropriate lifestyle changes known to improve estrogen metabolism, including taking supplements, increasing exercise, and eating more cruciferous vegetables. If we improve her estrogen profile, we then help her reach a decision about BHRT based on her individual risk factors and needs. For example, if she has no risk factors for breast cancer and is rapidly losing bone mass, we may decide that it's worth the risk to prescribe hormones to preserve her bones, especially during the first five years of postmenopause, when bone loss is the greatest. But we continue to carefully monitor her estrogen metabolites and her clinical course.

After administering BHRT, we redo the hormone metabolite test to make sure that she is not producing excess bad estrogens. If, despite our best efforts, she is still overproducing bad estrogens and has other significant risk factors, we may discontinue BHRT.

The one thing to remember is that there are no absolutes in medicine. One woman could make a preponderance of bad estrogen metabolites for many years and never get cancer. Another woman with a more predisposed body may get cancer even with lower exposures. We believe that as long-term studies of this approach to breast cancer prevention become available in the future we will be able to counsel our patients with greater precision.

## HORMONE OPTIONS

BHRT is available in predosed pharmaceutical preparations, which are sold at your local drug store by prescription, or as individually dosed hormones prepared by a compounding pharmacist based on your physician's *specific* prescription for you. There are hundreds of compounding pharmacies in the United States. If you don't live near one, you can fill a prescription by mail. If you've never used a compounding pharmacist, there is nothing new or unusual about them. At one time, most prescriptions in the this country were filled by compounding pharmacies, but today, most drugs come predosed and prepackaged. The prepackaged drug method of practicing medicine may enable doctors to see many more patients in this era of managed care, but it may not be the best medicine for all patients, especially in prescribing hormones.

Depending on your goal for BHRT, one treatment approach may work better for you than the other. If your goal is simply symptomatic relief, and you plan to get off hormones as soon as possible, the predosed hormones are probably fine for you. As a rule, your doctor will prescribe the lowest dose possible to relieve your symptoms. Furthermore, not every doctor is knowledgeable in dosing hormones or is comfortable working with a compounding pharmacist. Some doctors prefer prescribing the pharmaceutical products we list on page 199, which work well for many women. Even so, there is little reason for a doctor to prescribe synthetic estrogen. If you are using hormones for perimenopausal and postmenopausal issues, make sure that your doctor knows that you want only bioequivalent hormones.

If your goal is to restore hormones back to more youthful levels to stave off aging, and you plan to stay on hormones for as long as you can, you should consider finding a physician who can tailor the prescription just for you. You don't want to be overdosed, nor do you want to be underdosed. You need to find a physician who can prescribe the right hormone combinations so you can enjoy all the benefits of BHRT at the lowest known risk.

BHRT is available in many different forms: pills, creams, gels, transdermal patches, vaginal suppositories, and subcutaneous implanted pellets. Each hormonal delivery system has its pros and cons. Depending on how many hormones you take, you may need to use more than one product.

Progesterone, testosterone, and estradiol can be included in the BHRT prescription if needed.

## Pills

Studies show that taken orally, non-bioequivalent hormones (specifically synthetic estrogen combined with progestin, synthetic progesterone) can stimulate the production of clotting factors, increasing the risk of blood clots. Even though bio-equivalent hormones may be safer than synthetic hormones when taken orally, we tend to prefer non-oral forms of BHRT.

The one exception to the rule is natural progesterone, an example of which is Prometrium, a micronized form of bioequivalent progesterone, which can be taken orally. Prometrium may actually protect against blood clots.

Many physicians agree that oral progestins (Provera, synthetic progesterone) should be avoided because of the increased risk for blood clots and breast cancer. Testosterone is rarely prescribed in pill form because of potentially dangerous side effects.

## Creams and Gels

Creams and gels deliver hormones through the skin. Hormone creams and gels are usually massaged into the chest, back, or trunk. Hormone creams and gels can be estrogen only, including a combination of estrogens (estradiol, estriol, and estrone) and natural progesterone, or testosterone. Many women choose to use estrogen creams and take oral progesterone.

These products are easy to use (unlike pellets, which must be inserted by a physician.) Creams and gels can be specifically dosed to individual patients and prepared by compounding pharmacies, or available in predosed pharmaceutical preparations sold in most stores. These products are a good choice for women looking for symptomatic relief because they tend to deliver lower levels of hormone than do other methods.

Progesterone creams are sold over the counter in many pharmacies and health food stores. As a rule we don't recommend using them because we don't think that a woman should use hormones unless she is under a doctor's care, and because most of these products may be too weak to have any real impact on her symptoms.

Even prescription-strength creams and gels are often inconsistently absorbed by the body, making it difficult to consistently achieve the right levels of hormones.

They can be messy and must be used daily or even twice daily. Creams and gels in particular can produce a weak hormonal response. If you are only looking for symptomatic relief and you have mild symptoms, these products may work well for you. Women who have taken artificial hormone pills that have powerful hormone-like effects are often disappointed if they switch to creams or gels. They do better on patches or pellets, which deliver a stronger and more consistent level of hormones.

One of the problems with creams and gels is that over time they can become temporarily ineffective. Your skin can develop what some call dermal fatigue syndrome and simply stop absorbing enough of the particular cream or gel. Although this syndrome has not been fully validated with proper research, we have seen it in our practice. If this happens, you may need to stop using the cream or gel for a while, change to a different formulation, or use a different method of BHRT.

## Vaginal Suppositories

Estrogen creams (estradiol) applied directly to the vagina are used primarily to prevent dryness and thinning of the vaginal wall. They are considered to be safe for most women; however, some estrogen is absorbed into the bloodstream. These creams may not be appropriate for some women with estrogen-dependent cancers or other risk factors.

## Transdermal Skin Patches

The most popular form of BHRT today combines an estradiol patch with oral progesterone (i.e., Prometrium). Hormone patches can be attached to the hip, lower back, or trunk and must be changed weekly or monthly.

Patches are easy to use and deliver a fairly consistent level of hormones in a natural way. Unlike creams, patches usually entail less dermal fatigue syndrome. Although skin patches may offer a more consistent level of hormones, they are not always as effective as pellets and can cause local irritation at the point of adhesion.

## Pellets

Many of our patients opt for hormone pellets (testosterone and estrogen, not progesterone) because they are very easy to use and highly effective. The pellet is about the size of a grain of rice. For women, we typically include an estradiol pellet and a testosterone pellet if needed. (We prescribe natural progesterone in pill form.) The hormones are tightly compressed within the pellet and are gradually absorbed into the bloodstream as the body needs them. The pellet bypasses the liver, reducing the risk of blood clots. The pellet is implanted under the skin in a five-minute office procedure.

Once the pellet is implanted, it is virtually worry free. Most people can go between four and six months before needing a new pellet. For some women, the pellet works better than other hormone delivery systems at providing a good consistent level of hormones. This route is especially preferred for women who want a longer-term solution to hormone deficiency. In our clinical experience, the pellet is the most effective way to bring FSH levels back to normal, which is a sign that the body is receiving a physiologic dose of estrogen; this is important for some but not all women. We find that other forms of BHRT—creams, gels, and the patch—do not restore FSH to premenopausal levels.

The downside is that physicians must receive special training to administer pellets, and therefore they are not widely available in the United States.

However, it has consistently been our experience that once women and men try the pellets, they usually never want to go back to the transdermal systems.

### HER

*"My husband and I are both doing bioequivalent replacement. Before he started on testosterone, he was always tired, and sexual intercourse was difficult. After he had his hormone levels checked, we discovered that his testosterone was very low for a man his age. He had testosterone pellets implanted. He had an immediate return of physical strength, and things corrected themselves in the bedroom.*

*I'm nearing menopause, and while I was having other blood work done I had my hormone levels checked. Dr. Bazzan found that my estrogen levels were dropping, so I decided to start BHRT. I take estrogen and testosterone now. It was a blessing. I never had to go through any of the terrible symptoms women my age go through. My feeling is, why go through it if you don't have to? And I'm hoping it keeps me feeling young."*

## Are You Getting the Right Dose?

The beauty of using bioequivalent hormones is that they can be dosed fairly accurately to each patient. If the first prescription doesn't relieve symptoms properly, we can change the dose and monitor hormone levels until we get it right. It all depends on what the patient wants and needs.

If a woman finds that she is not getting the right dose to relieve her symptoms, we retest her and possibly might need to increase the dose or switch her to a different form of BHRT.

Many of our patients, however, are taking BHRT not only to relieve symptoms but to prevent or reverse osteoporosis and other age-related ailments. In such cases, we believe that it is necessary to restore key hormones to their youthful levels.

## BHRT AT YOUR LOCAL PHARMACY

A wide range of pharmaceutical, predosed, bioequivalent
hormone products are available at most pharmacies.
Below is a list of common brands.

### FOR WOMEN

*Estrogen*
Oral
Estrace 17 (beta-estradiol)
0.5 mg, 1.0 mg, 2.0 mg

Ortho-Est (estropipate, estrone)
0.75 mg, 1.5 mg

Ogen (estropipate, estrone)
0.75 mg, 1.5 mg

Transdermal Estrogens
Estraderm (estradiol)
0.05 mg, 0.1 mg

Vivelle (estradiol)
0.035 mg, 0.05 mg
0.075 mg, 0.1 mg

Alora (estradiol)
0.05 mg, 0.075 mg, 0.1 mg

Climara (estradiol)
0.025 mg, 0.05 mg
0.075 mg, 0.1 mg

FemPatch (estradiol)
0.025 mg

### FOR MEN

Topical Testosterone
AndroGel 1% gel
1 pack delivers
2.5 mg over 24 hours
1 patch delivers
5 mg over 24 hours

Testoderm
1 patch delivers
4 mg over 24 hours
1 patch delivers
6 mg over 24 hours

Androderm
1 patch delivers
2.5 mg over 24 hours
1 patch delivers
5 mg over 24 hours

**FOR WOMEN (CONT'D)**

Esclim (estradiol)
0.025 mg, 0.0375 mg,
0.05 mg, 0.075 mg, 0.1 mg

Vaginal Estrogens
Estrace cream (estradiol)
0.1 mg

Ogen cream (estradiol)
1.5 mg/gm
Vagifem (estradiol vaginal tablets)
25 mcg in single-use applicator

*Progesterone*
Oral

Prometrium oral micronized
progesterone
100 mg, 200 mg
Vaginal Suppository
Crinone natural progesterone
4% (45 mg progesterone)
8% (90 mg progesterone)

Estrogen/Testosterone
Oral Estratest h.s. (esterified estrones)
0.625/1.25 mg
(methyltestosterone)
Estratest
1.25/2.5 mg

Testosterone for men is available in
pharmaceutical, predosed products

## THE YAM SCAM

Wild yam cream is sold in health food stores and pharmacies as a treatment for menopausal symptoms. Manufacturers would have you believe that when you rub the cream on your skin, it is absorbed by the body and converted into progesterone. This simply isn't true. The human body cannot convert wild yam cream into progesterone or any other hormone. The actual conversion of wild yam into an actual hormone is a chemical process that must be done under the right conditions in a laboratory. Don't waste your money on these creams!

# HIS HORMONE MAKEOVER

**HIM**

*"I can't tell you the impact that testosterone replacement has had on my life. It's been a quantum leap in terms of stamina, overall well-being, and feeling healthy. I feel now like I did in my late 30s, and I'm not exaggerating. When I was in my early 30s, I had this strong passion to work hard, play hard, and do other things with a passion. By my late 40s, I was tired all the time. Within a week of receiving the pellets for the first time, I felt like an entirely different person in terms of stamina and strength. A side benefit, which I'm never going to complain about, is the sex benefit."*

When a middle-aged man complains of fatigue, loss of sex drive, and difficulty maintaining muscle mass no matter how much he works out, we have a pretty clear idea what's wrong with him before we even get him into an examining room. He is suffering from the telltale signs of testosterone deficiency, sometimes referred to as *andropause.*

Of course, before we make a definitive diagnosis, we run the requisite tests to rule out other serious health problems, and we also order a hormone panel to measure his hormone levels. Very often, testosterone deficiency is not his only problem; low levels of this key male hormone often go hand in hand with obesity, heart disease, diabetes, and even depression.

Testosterone in men is a marker of both health and longevity. Young men with low testosterone levels have many of the same problems seen in much older men, such as loss of bone, poor muscle mass, excess body fat, poor sexual function, and depression. Low testosterone in midlife men seems to be a sign of accelerated aging.

Recent studies suggest that low testosterone levels can shorten a man's life. Since the 1970s, researchers in the Department of Family and Preventive Medicine at the University of California, San Diego School Medicine, have been observing 800 men, ages 50 to 91, who were living in Rancho Bernardo, California. At the beginning of the 1980s, researchers found that about one-third of the men in the study had lower than normal blood testosterone levels for their age group. Over the next 18 years, men with lower testosterone had a 33% greater risk of death than the group with normal testosterone levels. These findings were recently reported in the *Journal of Clinical Endocrinology and Metabolism.*

The study showed that men with low testosterone were more likely to have high levels of inflammatory cytokines, elevated markers for inflammation—a contributing if not causal factor for most chronic diseases. Clearly, low levels of testosterone should be taken seriously as a sign of a potential health threat. More important, low testosterone levels can interfere with a man's ability to function to his full potential in the bedroom, at the gym, and even at work.

Testosterone is the primary male hormone, but men also produce small amounts of DHEA, estrogen, and progesterone. After age 30, men gradually lose about 1% to 2% of their testosterone every year. Depending on how much a man starts out with, this loss can be minimal, or it can be devastating. In some cases, the testosterone-estrogen balance can be thrown off, and this can cause some nasty side effects such as gynecomastia (male breasts), loss of body hair, and big bellies.

Abdominal obesity, a virtual epidemic today, is particularly bad news for men who care about maintaining their testosterone levels. Fat cells contain an enzyme called aromatase, which converts testosterone into estradiol, the metabolites of which may be a factor in promoting benign prostate hypertrophy (BPH) and even prostate cancer. Abdominal fat cells are particularly aggressive in terms of "feminizing" testosterone, and men with big bellies often have abnormally high levels of estrogen and low levels of testosterone.

Hence, testosterone deficiency is often a result of an unhealthful lifestyle. Poor diet, lack of exercise, and too much stress can interfere with testosterone production, and a big belly can turn testosterone into estrogen. Since testosterone levels drop naturally in midlife men, these lifestyle factors make a bad situation even worse.

We're not suggesting that all men need testosterone replacement. If you have normal levels of testosterone, testosterone replacement therapy is not going to do much for you. If you have low levels of testosterone, however, restoring them to normal will make you feel better and improve your body composition. We want to point out that we don't advocate using testosterone-boosting drugs to improve performance, as some athletes have been known to do. The normal physiologic doses we recommend are not going to turn you into a superman. The drugs that rev up your testosterone to unhealthy levels can be very dangerous. At any age, taking testosterone when you don't need it is putting yourself at unnecessary risk.

As more and more baby-boomer men reach their 50s and 60s, testosterone replacement therapy is growing in popularity. Unlike HRT for women, testosterone therapy was never as widely prescribed to men, but it is starting to catch up.

## THE PHYSICAL EXAM FOR MEN

Before we prescribe BHRT to a man, we first do a complete history and physical examination to (1) make sure he is in good health, (2) determine if he is a good candidate for hormone replacement, and (3) tailor a prescription to meet his needs. As with women, we ask men to fill out a detailed questionnaire about his health and lifestyle. We base our treatment recommendations on the test results, the questionnaire, and our patient interview.

What tests should men have, and when should they have them? Below, we offer our general guidelines for medical tests for men based on age and risk factors. Your physician may recommend additional tests or more rigorous follow-up, based on your family or medical history.

# PREVENTIVE HEALTH EXAM

At age 20, everyone should have a complete fasting lipid profile performed every five years. If you have a lipid imbalance, your doctor may require this test to be done more frequently.

Starting at age 40, everyone should have a comprehensive physical examination, including a detailed family medical history, all basic lab tests, a blood pressure check, and a review of potential risk factors.

Height and weight should be taken at each visit and carefully monitored. The basic preventive health exam should be repeated at least every three years until age 50.

Starting at age 50, it should be done every two years. And by age 65, it should be done annually. After age 65, vision and hearing should be checked annually as part of the exam.

## Diabetes Screen

All men with high blood pressure or dyslipidemia (bad blood fats) should be given a fasting plasma glucose test to screen for diabetes.

## Colon Cancer Screen

Starting at age 50, all men should have a colonoscopy every three to five years. After age 80, this test should be done at the discretion of the patient and the doctor.

## Prostate Cancer Screen

Starting at age 50, men should talk to their physicians about having a prostate-specific antigen (PSA) test and a digital rectal exam (DRE). The need for the tests depends on risk factors and symptoms. Men over 65 are at a higher risk for cancer and could be even harboring a latent cancer. Before starting testosterone replacement therapy, they should have a detailed discussion with both their primary physician and a urologist about further testing. A biopsy of the prostate is the most accurate diagnostic test for cancer.

### Abdominal Aortic Aneurysm Screen

Between the ages of 65 and 75, all men who have *ever* smoked should have a one-time abdominal ultrascreen for a possible abdominal aortic aneurysm.

### Baseline Bone Density Test

We also recommend a bone density test (DEXA scan) for men over 80 or any man with an increased risk of bone loss because of chronic diseases or treatments that hurt the bones

### Check Levels of Key Hormones

#### FSH

FSH levels can be too low or too high, depending on the problem. In the case of primary hypogonadism, testosterone levels are low, and FSH (and LH) are elevated. This is an indication that the testicles are not making enough testosterone, causing the surge in FSH and LH.

In the case of secondary hypogonadism, the pituitary itself does not produce enough FSH and LH, and the testicles have no feedback guidance, which means that FSH (and LH) will be low or normal.

#### ESTRADIOL

High levels of estradiol (estrogen) indicate a possible relative testosterone deficiency. Men with excess estrogen are at risk of producing the potent form of estrogen that is carcinogenic—not to mention that they can have some nasty side effects, like enlarged breasts, poor muscle tone, and fatigue.

### TESTOSTERONE, TOTAL AND FREE

Most testosterone is bound to a protein called sex-hormone-binding globulin (SHBG) and is released into the bloodstream as needed. That's why just measuring total testosterone doesn't tell the real story about how much testosterone is actually available for the body to use. In reality, only a very small amount of total testosterone in the body is free, or unbound, testosterone. As men age, the amount of testosterone on SHBG increases, leaving less testosterone for use.

### DHT

DHT (dihydrotesterone) must remain in physiologic levels. It is 1.5 to 2.5 times more potent than testosterone, and too much can create problems with prostate cancer and male-pattern baldness.

### TSH

Elevated levels of thyroid-stimulating hormone could indicate a thyroid problem, which can affect the male reproductive system. Thyroid dysfunction can be associated with ED. If necessary, we prescribe thyroid medication.

### SHBG

As mentioned earlier, most of the testosterone in the body is bound to SHBG and is released into the bloodstream as the body needs it. Elevated levels of SHBG suggest that not enough free testosterone is available to the body.

## HORMONE OPTIONS

Most testosterone prescriptions are written for bioequivalent forms of the hormone. Like BHRT for women, they are available in predosed pharmaceutical preparations and sold by prescription at most pharmacies, or they can be individually dosed by compounding pharmacists based on your doctor's prescription.

In our practice, testosterone is not given orally because it is metabolized by the liver and can cause severe acne, as well as other negative and potentially dangerous side effects. Testosterone can also be administered by injection, but now that there are so many effective testosterone products on the market, this method is not used as often.

### Creams and Gels

Testosterone gel is the most commonly prescribed form of this hormone in the United States. It's available by prescription at most pharmacies and discount drug stores. Both creams and gels can be individually dosed for each patient by a compounding pharmacist based on a doctor's prescription.

You must use the cream or gel once or twice daily at about the same time each day to maintain a consistent level of hormone. Creams and gels are usually applied to the upper arms, chest, or abdomen. These products are easy to use and work well for many of our patients. Within a few weeks, testosterone levels return to normal, and men feel more like themselves again.

Some men don't like handling creams or gels because they can get messy. As with anything you put on your skin, there is a possibility of skin irritation. And as with any skin preparation, there is a risk of variability in absorption.

### Transdermal Skin Patch

An adhesive patch containing testosterone is attached to the skin, but it must be changed daily or weekly, depending on the product. Patches are available in pre-dosed pharmaceutical preparations that are sold by prescription at most pharmacies, or they can be individually dosed by compounding pharmacists based on a doctor's prescription.

Patches should be placed on areas of skin with good blood supply and no hair (ouch!), such as the shoulders or the torso.

The testosterone patch is widely available and easy to use, but the adhesive on the patch can cause local skin irritation. Some men don't like the bother of having to change the patch daily.

## Pellets

A pellet about the size of a grain of rice is implanted under the skin in a five-minute procedure, using local anesthesia. Each pellet contains up to 200 milligrams of crystalline testosterone. Depending on the patient, the total dose can usually be from 600 to 1,500 milligrams. This dosage allows the treatment to last between four and six months for most men. Testosterone is slowly released into the body, very much like the hormones that are naturally produced.

Once pellets are implanted, most men can go between four and six months before needing new pellets. Testosterone levels stay fairly consistent until the pellets run out. We regard the slow-release pellets as the Cadillac of BHRT. They're not available everywhere in this country, but of all forms of BHRT, they are the easiest to use and most effective in restoring hormones back to their normal levels if you have the option.

There is a downside. Physicians must receive special training to administer pellets, and that limits their availability in United States. And unlike patches, creams, and gels, which patients can replenish on their own, new pellets must be implanted by your doctor every four to six months. This entails an extra visit to the doctor's office as well as additional cost.

Every decision about BHRT, for either women or men, must be made carefully, on an individual basis, after careful analysis of the patient's medical history, symptoms, and personal requirements. There are no shortcuts in patient care. We hope that this chapter provides you with the background you need to make an informed, intelligent decision with your doctor.

## CHAPTER TEN

# SUPPLEMENT MAKEOVER

We strongly believe that good nutrition is the foundation of a healthful lifestyle. There is simply no substitute for the right diet. Under ideal conditions, most vitamins and minerals should be obtained by eating fresh fruits and vegetables. There are literally thousands of beneficial chemicals in food (phytochemicals) that have yet to be studied, and their potential is vast. When we isolate a particular vitamin or food extract and make it into a pill, we may be missing out on other important phytochemicals that nature intended for us to eat.

For example, when you eat an orange, you're not just getting ascorbic acid, the vitamin C that you find in most vitamin pills. You're also getting a full range of citrus bioflavonoids, which not only aid in the absorption of vitamin C in the body but provide unique health benefits of their own. Although a multivitamin may contain vitamin C complex with bioflavonoids, we believe that the quality and bioavailability (how well it's absorbed by the body) of these nutrients is better in the original fruit.

As we tell our patients, *the wrong diet cannot be fixed by the right supplements.* We recognize, however, that it is not always possible to eat well every day, as hard as we may try. Even people who eat well may not be getting enough of some key nutrients that are hard to find in food. In these situations, supplements can help fill the nutritional gap.

There are thousands of supplements on the market, and it can be very confusing—if not overwhelming—for the average person to try to sort through all those products. You don't need to take a lot of supplements to achieve optimal health, but you do need to take the right ones. To make it simple, we recommend a *limited* group of supplements for both men and women to take every day.

## TAKE A MULTIVITAMIN DAILY

First, we believe that everyone should take a *comprehensive multivitamin* daily. Why? There are some essential nutrients that we need in higher amounts than are normally available in food. In addition to containing adequate vitamins and minerals, your multivitamin should also contain enzymes that facilitate the absorption of nutrients as well as phytonutrients, helpful chemicals found in plants that you may not be able to get in your food even if you eat lots of fruits and veggies.

It's not uncommon for people in their middle years and beyond to be taking one or more drugs, whether prescription or over the counter. What you may not know is that many medications can deplete the body of important nutrients, and this can result in nutrient deficiency. For example, every time you pop an antacid, take medication to lower your blood pressure, or use oral contraceptives, you could be depleting some of your B vitamins. Not only are B vitamins good for mood, well-being, and heart health, but they are essential in driving the reactions inside the mitochondria of all cells, which create the energy that runs the body.

You may be surprised to learn that the right diet enriched by supplements can also help to overcome bad genetics. Many people mistakenly believe that they can't do anything about their genes. This simply is not true.

We all carry our fair share of good genes and bad genes. But here is the big news: they are not carved in stone. More precisely, genes have the potential to *express* (behave) differently in different situations. There are different versions of the same gene, called *polymorphisms*. The good or bad version of the same gene is activated by the person's lifestyle. That may seem complicated, but it helps explain what makes us unique. And it helps explain why it's possible for one brother to gorge on bad food and get away with it while the other watches every morsel and can still get into trouble.

An unhealthful lifestyle—smoking, being sedentary, eating poorly, and exposure to toxins—can turn on bad versions of the genes. The good news is that the reverse is also true: The right lifestyle can turn on good genes and turn off bad genes, and the effect can be especially powerful when combined with the right supplements. For example, the three supplements that we call estrogen tamers (see page 220) can help reduce the ill effects of bad cancer-causing estrogens.

Below, we review the select group of supplements that we recommend for men and women over 40 who want to achieve optimal health. These supplements have strong scientific backing and offer a wide range of benefits. We have designed a brand of supplements that we offer our patients and can be obtained on our Web site, www.greatlifemakeover.com. We did this to ensure that our patients were using the highest quality supplements, but you can purchase other brands of the supplements listed below at most health food stores, in pharmacies, and on the internet. We urge you to stick to reputable manufacturers who offer products that have been vetted by third-party testers, to make sure that you're actually getting what you pay for. We are pleased to note that more and more physicians are prescribing supplements for their patients. Of course, you need to inform your doctor about any supplements you may be taking on your own. Some supplements can interact with medications or may need to be discontinued before surgical procedures.

## FOR EVERYONE AT 40 PLUS

### Probiotics

Your gut is home to more than 100 *trillion* different microscopic organisms, including hundreds of different species of "good" bacteria, such as *Lactobacillus acidophilus, L. bulgaricus,* and *B. bifidum,* among others. There are actually more bacteria living inside your body than the number of human cells that make up your body. They are there for a reason. Good bacteria perform many crucial jobs. They are essential for digestion and the function of the immune system; they work with the liver to protect the body from toxins; they help control the growth of bad bacteria, fungi, and yeast; and they produce many vitamins, including vitamin K.

Probiotics are best known for their impact on gastrointestinal health. Doctors often advise patients to supplement with a probiotic when they take an antibiotic, because as the drug is killing the harmful bacteria that are causing the infection, it is also killing the good bacteria in the gut that are keeping us healthy and are protective against disease. Recent research suggests that probiotics may have anticarcinogenic and tumor suppression effects, as well as control inflammation and even help with weight loss. They also help to favorably modulate the function of the immune system.

As we age, good bacteria tend to die off. Stress, exposure to toxins (especially antibiotics), and poor diet can accelerate the loss of good bacteria. That's why we recommend that everyone take a probiotic, a supplement containing live cultures of good bacteria. Although good bacteria are added to yogurt and other so-called health foods, these organisms may not be numerous enough; also, they are fragile and easily destroyed. On the basis of our clinical experience, we don't believe that enough active cultures may remain in these foods to be effective. Furthermore, as you may know by now, we're not crazy about dairy products to begin with, so we recommend that you use a nondairy source for your probiotic that contains high numbers of living cultures.

## Omega-3 Fatty Acids
### DOSE

Take 2,000 to 3,000 milligrams of omega-3 fatty acids daily.

Omega-3s are essential fatty acids—*essential* is the operative word. Your body needs good fat—and this good fat in particular—to run at optimal levels. Omega-3 fatty acids are a major component of cell membranes, the protective coverings that encase all of the trillions of cells in your body. Cell membranes are the gatekeepers of the cells. They perform a myriad of functions, including allowing nutrients and other beneficial substances into the cell, and excreting the bad stuff. Cell membranes not only are important for the structural integrity of your body but are key to communication between cells.

In the body, omega-3 fatty acids from food are mainly broken down into two other fatty acids: eicosapentaenoic acid (EPA) and docosahexaenoic acid (DHA). There are high amounts of DHA in the brain, and low levels of this fat have been linked to depression, moodiness, and even Alzheimer's disease. Omega-3 fatty acids are also important for cardiovascular health and are probably one of the few supplements routinely prescribed by cardiologists! In 2002, the American Heart Association gave it its seal of approval for patients who have heart disease to take omega-3s as long as they do so under a doctor's supervision.

There are two types of essential fatty acids—omega-3 fatty acids and omega-6 fatty acids, which are found in cooking oils, nuts, and most seeds and cereals. We get a lot of omega-6 fats in our diet, but we often fall short on omega-3s. The problem is that omega-6 fatty acids in excess can be inflammatory, whereas omega-3 fatty acids are *anti*-inflammatory.

In sum, if you want your body to work well, you need to feed it enough omega-3 fats. Therein lies the problem.

Omega-3 fatty acids are found in cold-water fatty fish (salmon, tuna, mackerel, halibut, and sardines), nuts, pumpkin seeds, and some grains. It's difficult, however, to get enough omega-3 fatty acids from food alone. First, most of the omega-3 fat is concentrated in the skin of fish, which many people don't eat. Second, fish that are high in fat also tend to be high in mercury, a heavy metal that can kill brain cells and cause neurological problems. In fact, some fish are so high in mercury that the Food and Drug Administration recommends that pregnant women and children not eat them at all.

Finally, modern food processing techniques remove essential fatty acids from foods to extend their shelf life and instead add pro-inflammatory saturated fats and trans fats, which are not as fragile and create metabolic logjams in the cells. In fact, when trans fats enter the body, they become incorporated into the cell membranes, unfavorably changing their structures and making them hard and rigid. High amounts of trans fats are associated with an increased risk of heart disease.

To achieve the right balance between omega-6 and omega-3 fatty acids, we urge everyone—along with the right diet—to take an omega-3 fatty acid supplement. There are two possible sources of omega-3 supplements: fish oil or vegetarian sources. Most of the studies confirming the health benefits of omega-3s have been performed with fish oil. For this reason, we recommend that you use a supplement based on fish oil, but be sure it is certified by a third-party lab to have been purified of mercury and other possible toxins. Omega-3 fatty acids like those in fish oil are easily oxidized and can turn rancid if not handled properly by the manufacturer. (That's why food manufacturers remove them from processed food!) At home, store your fish oil capsules in a cool, dark place out of direct sunlight.

Flaxseeds are the primary source of omega-3 fatty acids for supplements used by vegans. Flaxseeds contain omega-3 fatty acids in a form that may not be as readily used by the body: alpha-linolenic acid, which is not as easy to convert into EPA, and DHA, the omega-3s commonly found in fish. A potential problem may be that some people are deficient in the delta-5 and delta-6 desaturase and the elongase enzymes necessary to make the conversion to the same fatty acids found in fish. Vegans can use the plant-based omega-3 supplements if they want to avoid any fish-based products, but we don't know whether they will be as effective as fish oil.

*Caution:* Omega-3 fatty acids are natural blood thinners, which can be problematic under certain circumstances. People who are taking coumadin, a blood thinner; or who will be undergoing surgery; or who have defibrillators should not take omega-3 supplements without the knowledge and careful supervision of their treating physicians.

## Carnitine
### DOSE
Take 500 to 1,500 milligrams daily.

Carnitine is an amino acid compound synthesized from the amino acids lysine and methionine. It's produced in the body, primarily in the liver and kidneys. It is concentrated in red meat and dairy products but is also present in vegetables, grains, wheat, and fruits. As we age, our production of carnitine declines, and it's difficult to make up the gap through diet alone, especially if we're eating a plant-based diet. As with omega-3 fatty acids, more and more doctors are recommending carnitine to their patients, mostly for its benefits to the heart, kidney, lipids, glucose metabolism, and brain. Gym rats have been using carnitine for years because they claim to feel benefits from it. Some studies have shown that it can improve aerobic ability and athletic performance, but others have not. And here's one for the guys—carnitine has been shown to improve sperm motility, which would increase the odds that sperm will fertilize an egg. Carnitine also may increase the androgen receptors and therefore the utilization and function of testosterone after exercise.

Carnitine is critical for the production of energy in the mitochondria, known as the energy-producing units, or "powerhouses" of the cell. Carnitine shuttles fatty acids across the mitochondrial membrane, where they are made into energy, and then helps to remove the waste products created by energy production in the mitochondria. This is very important because if toxic byproducts are allowed to accumulate in the mitochondria, they can damage them and slow down energy production.

Energy is absolutely essential to sustain life; without it, your body couldn't perform any of the tasks needed to keep you alive. As we get older our mitochondria begin to get less efficient and die off, which can leave our organ systems starved for energy. In fact, many scientists believe that the loss of mitochondria is a prime cause of aging, leaving us more vulnerable to heart disease, cancer, and Alzheimer's disease.

Cell studies and animal studies have shown that taking supplemental carnitine can repair damage in mitochondria and bring them back to a more youthful level of functioning. In fact, in animal studies, carnitine has been proved to be remarkable in terms of helping stave off the physical and mental signs of aging. There's tantalizing new evidence that this supplement may help reverse the signs of aging in humans. Italian researchers at the University of Catania wanted to see the effect of carnitine supplementation in adults 100 years old or older. At the beginning of the study, centenarians all suffered from impaired mobility, general weakness, decreased mental health, and poor endurance. Sixty-six men and women participated in the study, which was published in the *American Journal of Clinical Nutrition*. Half the group received 2 grams of carnitine daily; the other half received a placebo. At the end of six months, the carnitine users had shown improvements in several key areas: On average, they lost 1.6 kg of fat, while the placebo group gained 0.6 kg fat; they had an increase in muscle mass, and they scored higher on mental function tests.

There is no doubt that carnitine plays a key role in heart health. Carnitine has been shown in animal studies to help to normalize elevated triglycerides, a blood fat that is closely associated with metabolic syndrome and prediabetes. At the same time, carnitine can raise levels of the good HDL cholesterol necessary for removing bad LDL cholesterol from the body. For several decades, carnitine has been studied as a treatment for angina and heart disease in Italy, Sweden, and Japan. Carnitine may be especially helpful for coronary artery disease because it helps the heart use its limited oxygen supply more efficiently.

Carnitine provides much-needed fuel for an aging brain. It is converted into acetylcholine, a neurotransmitter that declines with age, and is essential for learning and concentration. As discussed in Chapter 3, "When You're Feeling Down," when we are under stress, our adrenal glands produce cortisol, a hormone that prepares the body to fight or flee. Our brain cells have special receptors that cortisol attaches to, signaling to the adrenal glands that it's time to stop producing it. But if we're constantly bombarding our brain cells with cortisol, the receptors will eventually become desensitized and can no longer provide the necessary feedback to the adrenal glands. So the adrenal glands just keep pumping out more and more cortisol. In animal studies, carnitine has restored cortisol receptors in aging animals. It makes sense that carnitine could do the same for humans and thereby improve the stress response.

## Coenzyme Q10

### DOSE

Take 60 milligrams daily.

Coenzyme Q10 (CoQ10) is a fat-soluble antioxidant made in the body. It was discovered in the 1960s and is best known for the critical role that it plays in energy production in the cells, specifically in the mitochondria. CoQ10 levels decline as we age. Some clinicians prescribe CoQ10 routinely to older patients on the assumption that it will reduce fatigue and improve health, and this makes sense to us.

Although there have been few studies of CoQ10 on healthy people, it has been well studied in clinical settings, specifically as a treatment for high blood pressure and heart failure as well as other conditions. It is often used along with conventional treatments for the treatment of ischemic heart disease, in which the heart is deprived of blood. CoQ10 inhibits the oxidation of cell membrane fats and fats circulating throughout the bloodstream. Studies have shown that CoQ10 helps bad LDL cholesterol resist oxidation, which is important because oxidized LDL can damage the arteries that deliver blood to the heart. Statin drugs, routinely prescribed to lower cholesterol, also decrease the production of CoQ10. Many physicians prescribe CoQ10 to their patients taking statin drugs. Mitochondrial dysfunction likely plays a role in migraine as well as in age-related visual problems, and therapies that include CoQ10 have been tried. The causes of several neurodegenerative disorders are very complex but partly involve impaired mitochondrial function and increased oxidative stress. CoQ10 acts both as an antioxidant and as an energy producer at the level of the mitochondria. In several animal models of neurodegenerative diseases, and in some human trials, CoQ10 has shown beneficial effects. CoQ10 appears to be safe and well tolerated, and several efficacy trials are planned.

CoQ10 may also help boost male fertility. Free radicals can damage sperm, just as they damage cells everywhere in the body. Studies have shown that in men with impaired sperm motility, CoQ10 supplementation increases the concentration of CoQ10 in seminal plasma and sperm cells and also improves sperm motility.

### Creatine

**DOSE**

Take 3,000 milligrams daily.

Studies show that a dose of 3 grams daily over approximately 4 weeks can significantly elevate muscle creatine concentration.

Some of you may be wondering, "Isn't this the supplement that athletes use? Why on earth should I take it?" For exactly the same reasons that they're taking it: to get the most out of your workout.

Creatine is made in the body from three amino acids: arginine, glycine, and methionine. We produce about 1 gram of creatine daily in the kidney and liver, and it is transported through the blood to the muscles. Creatine-containing foods are meat, fish, and poultry, which provide about 1 gram daily of creatine. Over 90% of the total body creatine is in skeletal muscle as free creatine and creatine phosphate (phosphocreatine).

Creatine builds stamina by helping your muscle cells recharge faster so that you can work out longer and harder. A vigorous workout depletes your muscles of creatine, which can be replenished by taking creatine supplements.

Many research studies and review papers support that creatine supplementation is ergogenic (has a positive effect on physical or mental performance) for short-term, high-intensity exercise gains in lean body mass and maximal muscle strength and weightlifting.

For those who are unfamiliar with creatine, rest assured that it's not in the same league as dangerous performance enhancement drugs—it is nonsteroidal and is considered safe for most people. It has become as common as protein powder in the locker rooms of amateur and professional athletes. According to the National Institutes of Health (NIH), about 25% of professional baseball players and 50% of all football players use creatine, making it the most popular sports supplement in the world. Creatine is also one of the most researched sports supplements in the world, and not just for its role in athletic performance. Creatine is being investigated as a treatment for a wide range of ailments, including bad blood lipids, the consequences of heart attack, and neuromuscular disorders.

Nor should women fear that creatine is going to make them "big" or "pumped." Creatine can't turn a woman into a muscle man any more than it can turn a man into one. On the other hand, with appropriate exercise, it may help both men and women maintain the muscle mass that is often lost during midlife.

Creatine should not be used with diuretics. Be sure to drink lots of water when you take creatine. Creatine should not be used by anyone with kidney or liver problems. Some people complain that creatine causes stomach upset, so if you find that you can't tolerate it, stop using it.

In sum, creatine won't make you stronger or leaner on its own, but it can help enhance your workout, and that will give you better results.

# FOR SPECIAL SITUATIONS

We recommend the following group of supplements to meet specific needs. They have less scientific evidence to support their use, and we are careful to underscore that when we discuss them with our patients. From our experience, they can be very helpful in terms of improving quality of life. And they meet our standards for safety—which is of course, of paramount importance.

### Hemp Seed Protein
**DOSE**
Drink up to three hemp shakes daily.

When you limit your intake of animal protein, you need to make sure that you are getting enough complete protein from other sources. If you fall short on protein, you may find that you are losing muscle even though you are working out. There are lots of protein products on the market, but most are dairy based, which we don't recommend. There are also soy-based proteins, but we prefer that you not overuse them. The jury is still out on whether soy can stimulate estrogen-based tumors, and until we know for sure, we don't advise the excess consumption of soy products. Some hemp products also have rice protein, which is fine.

Hemp seed is an easily digestible form of protein that contains a good balance of amino acids and is a good source of omega-3s.

The downside is that some hemp seed powder products are gritty and don't mix well. Using a blender can help create a good consistency. We particularly like Nature's Harvest, and we've gotten good feedback on it from our patients. Mix it with a low-sugar soy, almond, or rice milk.

The word "hemp" alarms some people because hemp comes from the same plant species as marijuana. There is a big difference—hemp contains only trace amounts of tetrahydrocannabinol (THC), the chemical that gives marijuana its psychoactive effects. The most popular brands (Living Harvest, Nutiva) guarantee that there is no THC in their products, and therefore you have no reason to be worried if you have to take a drug test.

## THREE SUPPLEMENTS TO TAME ESTROGEN

We routinely check both our male and our female patients for their levels of estrogen metabolites to determine whether they are prone to make cancer-causing "bad" estrogen (catechol estrogen metabolites) or "good" estrogen (methylated estrogen) that may protect against cancer. Several studies suggest that women with high levels of "bad" estrogen are at higher risk for breast cancer. Furthermore, in our clinical experience we have found that women who are loaded with bad estrogen tend to have the worst PMS and perimenopausal symptoms.

Men can also fall victim to the ill effects of bad estrogen, especially when their testosterone levels begin to decline. Testosterone can be converted into estrogen by aromatase, an enzyme found predominantly in fat cells. As men get older—and fatter—they may find that too much testosterone is being converted into estrogen, which can turn into bad estrogen metabolites. Bad estrogen may promote benign prostatic hypertrophy (BPH) and prostate cancer.

Although genetics plays a role in estrogen metabolism, so do diet and supplements. Many fruits and vegetables contain phytochemicals that can help improve estrogen metabolism, which could explain why people who eat plant-based diets have the lowest rates of cancer.

Three of these important phytochemicals are available in supplements: calcium-D-glucarate, diindolylmethane (DIM), and resveratrol. We recommend these three supplements to all men and women who are using BHRT to help lower bad estrogens and promote the production of good estrogen metabolites. On the basis of experience with our patients, we have found that these supplements can reduce bad estrogens in both men and women and may boost the level of free testosterone in men.

These supplements may interfere with the effectiveness of birth control pills, and women who are using oral contraception should avoid them.

Also, although we discuss potential cancer protective effects, there is no conclusive evidence on this, and we want to underscore that we do not see any supplements or diet as cancer treatment. *Once a cancer is diagnosed, conventional oncological care is necessary, and good nutrition is an adjunct to maintaining as much strength and vitality as possible during the cancer treatment process.*

### Calcium-D-Glucarate

**DOSE**

Take 400 to 1,200 milligrams daily for general detoxification.

Calcium-D-glucarate is the calcium salt of D-glucaric acid, a substance produced in the body and found in many fruits and vegetables, especially cruciferous vegetables, apples, oranges, and grapefruit. The human body metabolizes potentially toxic chemicals (including bad estrogen metabolites) in the liver by attaching detoxifying substances such as glucuronic acid to them and excreting them through bile in the intestine for elimination. The faster you can get rid of these toxins, the better. Calcium-D-glucarate blocks beta-glucuronidase, a dangerous enzyme in the body, which is produced by unfriendly bacteria in the gut. The beta-glucuronidase breaks the carefully crafted bond between glucuronic acid and these toxins. This is bad because it allows toxins and bad hormones to return into circulation from the gut and stay in the body longer. Usually this is unbeknownst to the person for many years. High levels of beta-glucuronidase are associated with an increased risk of breast, prostate, and colon cancer. Cell studies and animal studies have shown that Calcium-D-glucarate inhibits the growth of human mammary tumor cells grown in mice. Glucarate suppresses protein kinase C and induces transforming growth factor-beta in the mammary tumor cells, so it may possibly be protective against certain cancers. Although no large-scale studies have yet been performed in humans, it makes sense that this supplement could have a cancer-protective effect in humans.

## DIM

### DOSE

Take 200 mg daily for women and 400 mg daily for men.

Diindolylmethane (DIM) is a chemical found in cruciferous vegetables, like broccoli, cabbage, and Brussels sprouts. Those vegetables are the best source, but it is hard to eat enough of them.

The active and beneficial substances in cruciferous vegetables are absorbable diindolylmethane and its precursor, indole-3-carbinol (I3C). Significant amounts of DIM are found in cruciferous plants, while I3C (which is unstable and only transiently present during digestion) is the natural precursor to DIM.

There is some debate in the supplement world as to which is better to take, because of absorption and conversion issues. The data support both, but we lean toward DIM.

DIM helps convert estrogen into good estrogen metabolites, and it may increase the amount of free testosterone in men by blocking aromatase (from fat cells), which converts testosterone into estrogen. Cell studies and animal studies have shown that DIM can block the growth of estrogen-sensitive tumors. Although there is no evidence yet that it works in humans, we feel that it has potential to be protective against breast cancer and prostate cancer.

Interestingly, DIM has become a popular sports supplement because athletes and body builders believe that it helps burn fat and promote lean mass. Given the fact that it may boost levels of free testosterone, it's possible DIM could improve the muscle-to-fat ratio.

## Resveratrol
### DOSE
Take 100 milligrams daily.

Resveratrol is a nutrient found in red grapes, red wine, berries, peanuts, and Japanese knotweed (*Polygonum cuspidatum*.) In recent years, there's a been a lot of buzz about resveratrol after researchers at Harvard and MIT found that it can extend the life of yeast, worms, mice, fruit flies, and some fish—no small feat. It is believed that resveratrol activates an enzyme found in many living organisms (including humans) called SIRT1. The hypothesis is that SIRT1 can turn on the switch that triggers cell repair, so that instead of dying, old cells keep rejuvenating. Animal studies have shown that very low calorie diets can produce the same longevity effect. What's exciting about resveratrol is that it can extend the life of animals without starving them. The hope is that resveratrol will work as well for humans, and we recommend it to people who want that potential edge.

We don't know whether resveratrol will extend life or not, but that's not why we recommend it. What intrigues us about resveratrol is that laboratory studies have shown it to be a potentially anticancer compound that fights cancer at all three phases: initiation, promotion, and progression. As some of you may know, cancer doesn't happen overnight. It takes years to develop, and under ideal conditions, our bodies kill off cancer cells before they can spread. If resveratrol works as well in humans as it does in animals, it could prove to be a weapon against certain types of cancer, nipping it in the bud before it can cause trouble as well as everywhere else along the way. Even better, resveratrol is nontoxic, and it could have wonderful side benefits, like a longer life span.

Resveratrol may be helpful to counter the symptoms of menopause. It binds to estrogen receptors and produces estrogen-like effects in women, which may reduce hot flashes, mood problems, and osteoporosis; it is also cardioprotective.

Resveratrol is also being tested as a treatment for Type 2 diabetes and as a weight loss drug. Given all the promising science behind resveratrol, we feel comfortable recommending it as part of our daily supplement regimen for patients who are particularly vulnerable, based on the criteria described above.

## SUPPLEMENTS FOR SEXUAL HEALTH

People with very mild symptoms may require just a little help to cope with midlife sexual health issues. For these people, we have designed a combination supplement, one for men and one for women, that contains herbs, amino acids, essential fatty acids, and other ingredients that may help normalize hormones, relieve symptoms, and in some cases boost libido. We offer these supplements with the caveat that although they are generally regarded as safe (although true "safety" studies have not been done), the scientific support is limited, and the evidence is largely anecdotal. In fact, the evidence is more lacking for some of these compounds than for anything else we discuss. We have found, however, that for many men and women, they do the trick. We tell our patients who are reluctant to use drugs to try these supplements first and see if they work for them. We monitor patients closely for any potential side effects or problems, especially since most supplements are not closely regulated by the Food and Drug Administration. You can purchase our products online or look for similar products that contain some of these key ingredients. Most of these products are sold in combination formulas, not as separate supplements. *Follow the dosing recommendation on the bottle.*

***Caution:*** Despite hundreds—if not thousands—of years of use, most herbs have not been well researched, and we don't know all the details of how they actually work in the human body. Consult your physician before using any herb, especially if you have or are at risk for a hormone-dependent cancer, such as breast cancer or prostate cancer.

# PROSEXUAL SUPPLEMENTS FOR MEN

### Arginine

Before the debut of ED drugs in the 1990s, L-arginine was one of the few treatments we had for men with erectile problems. Arginine is an amino acid that boosts the body's production of nitric oxide, which improves blood flow to the penis and everywhere else. This should help a man get an erection and maintain it for a longer period of time. There is substantial anecdotal evidence that arginine improves sexual function in some but not all men. But then again, ED drugs work in only two-thirds of all men who use them. Body builders take arginine to enhance their workouts and promote muscle production. Studies have shown that arginine can stimulate the secretion of growth hormone by the pituitary gland. As we age, the production of growth hormone falls off, and this can affect muscle mass, cell repair, and bone density, among other things. Boosting growth hormone with arginine may prevent or reverse some of these changes. (There is anecdotal evidence that arginine may aggravate herpes outbreaks.)

### Tribulus terrestris

Also known as puncturevine, *Tribulus terrestris* is a herb that has long been used in traditional Indian (Ayuverdic) and Chinese medicine to treat depression, low libido, and related sexual problems. Today it is used to rev up male sex drive and as a sports supplement. A few studies have shown that it may increase pressure in the corpus cavernosum, which suggests that the erectile property of this herb could possibly result from an increase in androgen and subsequent release of nitric oxide from the nerve endings in the corpus cavernosum. Some other studies suggest that *Tribulus* may raise levels of luteinizing hormone (LH), which could boost testosterone levels; but again, the data are very limited.

## Epimedium Extract

This herb has been used in traditional Chinese medicine for hundreds of years as a tonic and sex enhancer. It is also known by the name horny goat weed because, according to legend, farmers noticed that after eating the weed their goats became more sexually active. It is thought that extracts of *Epimedium* relax the corpus cavernosum smooth muscle, thereby promoting erection through the effects on nitric oxide/phosphodiesterase type 5 (in an action similar to that of ED drugs). Furthermore, *Epimedium* has been shown to inhibit an enzyme known as acetylcholinesterase, which can interfere with sensory nerves, decreasing sexual desire and the ability to have an erection. (The same enzyme is involved in the promotion of Alzheimer's disease, another disease in which this herb is also being researched as a potential treatment.)

*Epimedium* appears to work best when combined with other herbs. It's also used by body builders because it's reputed to raise testosterone levels; this has been proved in animal studies but not in humans.

## Muira Puama

Known as potency wood, this Brazilian herb, *Ptychopetalum olacoides,* has been used as an aphrodisiac for centuries. Recent studies suggest that it may protect brain cells from oxidative damage, at least in mice. In 2000, at the Institute of Sexology in Paris, France, a clinical study with 202 women patients complaining of lack of sexual desire demonstrated muira puama extract to be effective. Within 4 weeks, 65% of patients with loss of libido claimed that the treatment was helpful. The institute is now planning a larger controlled study.

Muira puama contains free long-chain fatty acids, essential oils, plant sterols, coumarin, lupeol, and an alkaloid named muirapuamine.

Muira puama has been shown to relax the corpus cavernosum of the penis in rabbits, and it is speculated that it may have a similar effect in humans. It may block an enzyme known as acetylcholinesterase. Blocking the activity of this enzyme makes more acetylcholine available. Acetylcholine is a neurotransmitter, and it also can increase blood flow in the genitals.

One caveat: Muira puama in high doses can cause insomnia.

# PROSEXUAL SUPPLEMENTS FOR WOMEN

### Black Cohosh

Native to North America, this herb *(Cimicifuga racemosa)* is a traditional remedy for arthritis but in recent years has gained popularity as an alternative to hormone replacement therapy. It is one of the few natural treatments that is being studied by the National Center for Complementary and Alternative Medicine (NCCAM). Some but not all studies suggest that this herb can relieve menopausal symptoms, such as hot flashes, vaginal dryness, and night sweats. Similarly, some of our patients find that it's helpful, and others don't. The NCCAM Web site notes that the longest study conducted on black cohosh lasted for 6 months—not enough to determine its long-term safety.

### Maca

Native to Peru, this herb has recently become enormously popular among women looking for a nonhormonal way to relieve menopausal symptoms. Although scientific data on this use for maca are scarce, there is abundant anecdotal evidence. In particular, women claim that it improves their mental focus, mood, and energy. And yes, many claim that it improves libido, as was shown in men in a small study.

Maca is considered an *adaptogen,* a herb that helps the body adapt better to stress. Studies in mice suggest that it might increase sexual activity in both men and women.

### Muira Puama

You'll notice that this herb is also used for men to stimulate libido and improve erectile function. In women, muira puama is not used to rev up libido but to treat menopausal symptoms, which, as any woman will tell you, can make sex the furthest thing from her mind. For both men and women, muira puama is a tonic herb, which means that it's reputed to promote energy and relieve stress, though there is little scientific data of its purported effects.

## Damiana

Damiana is available in capsules, in extracts, and in dried leaves or powder to make a tea. The recommended doses for these commercial damiana products differ greatly, so follow directions on the package.

To make damiana tea, add 2 to 4 grams of dried leaves or leaf powder to about 8 ounces of boiling water. After it is allowed to stand for a few minutes, the mixture is strained to remove solids. Up to 3 cups of damiana tea may be consumed daily.

Damiana has been used as an aphrodisiac and a treatment for depression throughout Mexico, Central America, South America, and West Indies. It has long been used to stimulate sexual response in both women and men. It is reputed to have thermogenic properties, which means that it boosts metabolism and may be a mild stimulant, but there is little science to back up these claims.

## CHAPTER ELEVEN

# MOOD MAKEOVER

How do you treat a bad mood? It all depends on whom you ask.

A psychiatrist might say that the first step is to correct any glitches in the biochemistry of the brain that may be causing the problem, and that the best way to do this is with antidepressant drugs.

A psychologist would agree that there could be a biochemical link, but to really treat the bad mood, you need to get to the root cause. Was it triggered by job stress? Relationship problems? A recent loss?

An internist might say, wait a minute; before you start prescribing antidepressants, or sending someone to therapy, you'd better do a complete physical to rule out physical illness, like cancer or heart disease, which can be a trigger for depression.

An endocrinologist would say, don't forget to check for out-of-whack hormones.

A dietitian might say that the first step is to clean up the diet to see if a bad mood is being caused by nutritional deficiencies.

A fitness expert might say that a sedentary lifestyle is to blame.

As mind-body specialists, we agree with . . . all of the above.

*A true mood makeover must address all these issues*: brain chemistry, emotional issues, potential illness, hormones, diet, and fitness. All the things we have recommended until now—from diet, to relationship advice, to information on how to rebalance your hormones—are all components of a mood makeover.

There are times when we prescribe antidepressants, notably to patients who are in serious pain and possible imminent danger. If someone is stuck in a deep depression, we don't recommend self-medicating with over-the-counter herbs or other supplements. That person needs to get immediate and appropriate medical care.

It's a different story for mild mood problems. In these situations, we typically try lifestyle changes first. In most cases, they are quite effective. This is especially true for the "I'm so stressed out" and the "I don't feel like myself" complaints we often hear from our patients.

We have our own formula for beating the midlife blues. Ours is a multifaceted program that draws on existing therapies, but we simplify and streamline them for people with busy lives, who don't have a lot of time and who don't want to learn a lot of new jargon. It consists of simple breathing and relaxation exercises that won't take more than a few minutes a day, but it can be highly effective in reducing stress and boosting mood.

We also encourage you to stay connected with the things you love to do and the people you love to do them with. Having fun and enjoying a close intimate relationship with someone special is very life affirming.

## TAKE A BREATHER

Here's one of the easiest ways to de-stress your body and your mind. The funny thing is that you do it all the time, but most people tend to do it wrong.

We're talking about breathing, of course. But the trick is this: you have to do it correctly.

When our sympathetic nervous system is overcharged in fight or flight mode, we tend to take short, shallow breaths. Since many of us live under the yoke of chronic stress, our breathing reflects our stressed-out state.

Studies show that doing something as simple as changing your breathing patterns can help melt stress away and turn on the relaxation response. That term was first coined by Herbert Benson, M.D., director of the Benson-Henry Institute of Mind-Body Medicine at Harvard Medical School. In 1975, Dr. Benson helped mainstream the concept of mind-body medicine in his best-selling book *The Relaxation Response*. In his book he reported that patients who meditated regularly experienced positive changes in the body, including lower blood pressure, a decrease in heart rate, and reduced muscle tension. In the long run, he found that meditation helped produce a feeling of well-being and a reduction in anxiety.

Meditation is one of several ways to achieve the relaxation response. Deep breathing, which is a component of meditation, may produce similar results. In 2005, Dr. Richard Brown and Dr. Patricia Gerbarg of Columbia University analyzed several studies and concluded that deep yoga-style breathing is an effective treatment for stress-related disorders as well as for depression and anxiety.

Here's what you need to do to take advantage of this natural stress reliever.

Set aside at least two minutes for your breathing exercise. Five minutes is ideal, and if you have the time for more, that's great. Even two minutes is still enough time to get a good result. Within a few minutes of breathing correctly, you feel calmer and more focused.

We recommend that you take at least two Breathing Breaks daily; one in the morning and one later in the day. Some people may find it helps to reenergize them in the afternoon. Others may find it helps them wind down before bedtime. And there's no reason why you can't take three or more Breathing Breaks daily. See what works best for you.

Sit in a comfortable position. *Clear your mind. This is your time, your break. Don't let others intrude on your two-minute escape.*

*Take a deep breath in. Focus on your inhalation. Feel the air travel to your lungs and into your stomach. It is best to breathe with your nose if possible (both inhalation and exhalation). Fill your lungs, but do so comfortably; don't force the air.*

*Concentrate on releasing the breath. Feel the air traveling from your stomach up through your chest to your nose and out. It may be helpful to count four full seconds for the inhale and six for the exhale.*

*Keep breathing in and out rhythmically. Think about how your lungs are filling up with air with every breath. Feel your diaphragm contract and lower when you inhale, and release when you exhale. Breathe out completely, but not forcefully. Let the exhalation flow on its own.*

*Focus on what a deep breath really feels like. Notice how your muscles start to relax, and how the tension of the day evaporates into the air.*

*If your mind starts to wander, if you find yourself thinking unrelated or even stress-provoking thoughts ("What's going on at the office?") it's normal. Just reset your brain so that you're once again focused on your breathing.*

*At the end of two to five minutes or so, when you're down to your last three breaths, end each breath with a relaxing sigh or "Ahhh" sound. Also, some people like to exhale with a particular sound, such as the well-known "Om."*

Repeat the Breathing Break as often as you like! This is good for you and makes you feel good.

## SIMPLE STRETCHES TO DO ANYWHERE, ANYTIME

Muscles that are not used can stiffen and tense up, which is made even worse when you are in flight-or-fight mode. Furthermore, tense muscles trigger the production of inflammatory chemicals that can be damaging to your body. High levels of inflammation, in turn, can contribute to osteoarthritis, the wearing away of cartilage in the joints, and osteoporosis, the thinning of bone.

Being sedentary can be very stressful. Simply sitting all day at work can create muscle tension that triggers inflammation and poor circulation. Periodically, getting up from your chair and walking can help release tight muscle fibers. Gentle stretching is also a good way to help loosen up your muscles and deactivate the stress response.

Below are three stretches you can do on the go. Try to do them in the morning and the afternoon, or any time you've been sitting for a long time.

We also recommend our more comprehensive stretching program on page 156 that is part of our Midlife Workout.

### Relax Your Chest and Shoulders

*Stand up tall, with your feet shoulder-width apart and your hands clasped behind your back. Pull back with your hands and gently roll your shoulders back. Take three deep breaths, inhaling into the stretch, feeling the muscles release with the exhales.*

### Upper Body Stretch

*Stand up tall, with your feet shoulder-width apart and your hands at your sides. Reach your arms over your head, breathe in, and gently reach for the sky until you feel a nice stretch. Don't tug or force it. Just enjoy it. Hold for ten seconds while breathing deeply, and repeat three times. It may be more comfortable for you to do this stretch lying flat on the floor, especially if you have back or neck issues.*

### Loosen Your Hips

*Stand up tall, with your feet flat on he floor and your legs straddled about 2 feet apart. While keeping your stomach in and your pelvis tilted forward, keep widening your stance until you feel a good stretch in your butt, hips, and upper thighs. Don't overdo it! Remember to breathe and keep your back arched. Hold for ten seconds, and repeat three times.*

## MUSCLE AWARENESS

When we try to explain the muscle-tension-stress connection, people often ask, "How can I relax my muscles if I don't even realize that I'm tensing them?" That's a very good question. The truth is that many people carry their tension in their muscles, but they're unaware that they are doing it. They may wonder why their backs ache, why their joints hurt, and why they can't turn their necks anymore without feeling pain, but they don't realize that muscle tension is a possible culprit if not the major cause.

We prescribe a specific exercise to help people distinguish between a tense muscle and a relaxed muscle. We recommend that everyone do a muscle check periodically throughout the day to release the tension that is building inside.

You can do this one sitting right at your desk, or lying on the floor.

*Make a muscle with your biceps. Feel the tension in your arms, and then release them, letting them go limp. Feel the difference between tension and relaxation. Repeat twice.*

*Fold your arms across your chest, until you feel your chest tense up and contract. Then release it. Let your arms flop down to your sides. Feel the difference between tense and relaxed.*

*Pull your stomach muscles in. Hold them tight. Then release them and let the belly go soft.*

*Tighten your butt. Hold it for a few seconds, and then release.*

*Tighten your thigh muscles. Either tense them or squeeze them against your closed fists. Hold the squeeze, and then let your legs flop out.*

*Tighten your calf muscles by putting your feet in the tiptoe position. Hold the squeeze, and then let your legs relax.*

*Close your eyes. Make a big, exaggerated smile to tense up your face muscles. Then let it go, and feel the release.*

## MAKING PEACE

We all have to put up with annoying events and difficult people during the day; it's part of life. But we don't have to let these petty annoyances get the better of us. We don't have to dwell on them. It's important to take time out each day to clear your brain of negative thoughts, particularly about people who may be giving you grief.

After you've completed your two minutes of breathing and relaxation, take a few extra seconds and think about the person who is the source of your stress—a difficult boss, an uncooperative spouse, a sullen colleague or employee. When you think about that person, say to yourself, "May you be joyous, may you be healthy, may you be at peace, may you be at ease." What you're really saying is that you wish the person could be different, but you accept that he or she may not change. Then move on to thinking about something in life that brings you joy. Doing this can have an immediate stress-reducing effect by disconnecting you from negative stress and emotions, while you engage your positive emotional self. You may not change the person merely by thinking this way, but you may change the way you deal with him or her. It's important to learn how to systematically redirect your thoughts to things that give you peace and pleasure until you physically feel a good feeling replace a bad one. This helps you maintain perspective of what is truly important in life and deserving of your energy.

A tip for reinforcing this is to take a moment to feel gratitude for the good things in your life. The attitude of gratitude is exceedingly healthful, and it provides balance to the stressful thoughts about achieving the next task or goal.

## MOOD BOOSTER FOR COUPLES

Here's a daily exercise that requires nothing more than kindness. Every day, write down three things that you like about your spouse and your relationship. The simple practice of setting these good thoughts to paper helps reduce symptoms of depression and anxiety. Feel free to share your positive thoughts with your spouse.

## PAY ATTENTION TO THE PRESENT

Some of our approach to meditation is based on mindfulness, a concept popularized by Jon Kabat-Zinn that has been systemized into a formal stress reduction program called mindfulness-based stress reduction (MBSR). Our clinic offers Kabat-Zinn's program, and we recommend his books such as *Full Catastrophe Living* and *Wherever You Go, There You Are* to our patients. Mindfulness is essentially learning to pay attention in the present moment and to observe the present moment without a good or bad judgment of it. Essentially, we create the space to look at "what is," which affords us the opportunity to better choose our reaction to it. To enhance observation of the moment, basic relaxation and meditative exercises are taught, some of which are grounded in basic principles of hatha yoga.

We like to apply some of these basic techniques to foster paying attention to the ongoing tapes in our heads. By "tapes" we mean what we are telling ourselves all the time. We recommend that at the end of the work day you write down the main things that felt good or bad about the day, and what you were telling yourself about those things. (For example, "If I don't write this brief perfectly, it will be the end of the world," or "I sounded like a jerk at that meeting.") This type of task allows the logical part of your brain to observe how the emotional part of the brain is reacting. It helps facilitate greater interaction between these often disconnected parts of your brain, which can open up all kinds of opportunities for change. The more you do this exercise, the better you get at it.

If you're not comfortable expressing yourself with the written word, try drawing, sketching, or painting as a means to communicate your thoughts and feelings. The point is to increase your awareness of the present moment, which facilitates the observation and paves the way for new insights and expanded choices for coping.

This approach is useful because it helps you understand what is stressing you out in your daily life and gives you a mode of expressing and observing it. Moreover, it helps you to recognize a truly Great Life and adhere to the makeover formulas for better health and well-being. Every day you have an opportunity to make better choices for a better life. For example, you know that the best snacks are the ones we suggest, such as our trail mix or a soy yogurt. Yet, consistently at midday, you ignore what you know—and, more important, what you really *want* to do— and instead eat a bag of cookies. While increased mindfulness may not be the total solution, it might be an important step in identifying an unhelpful script ("I need these cookies to offset the pain of my job") and allowing the observing part of the brain to step and in and offer other options to offset the pain. Perhaps your observing brain could come up with something even more pleasurable that you know is a real treat to your physiology, like a ten-minute chair massage at a local spa. At the end of the massage, you'll feel refreshed, but you won't feel defeated or guilty about giving in to cravings. And you'll be happier and healthier for it.

## A PLUG FOR OUR WORKOUT

Exercise is a proven way to reverse a bad mood. In fact, a growing body of scientific literature confirms that exercise is a powerful antidepressant. Moderate but consistent exercise can have a positive impact on your brain chemistry that rivals that of widely prescribed psychotropic drugs.

A groundbreaking study conducted at Duke University in 1999 and published in the *Archives of Internal Medicine* compared three different forms of therapy to treat major depression in 156 men and women over the age of 50. One group was put on a program of aerobic exercise alone, another group was given antidepressants alone, and a third group was given a combination of aerobic exercise with antidepressants for 16 weeks. The researchers concluded that although the antidepressants worked faster, exercise worked well too, but it took longer. They recommended that "an exercise training program may be considered as an alternative to antidepressants for treatment of depression in older persons." Of course, another benefit is that exercise doesn't have any of the negative side effects of antidepressants, including delayed sexual response and possibly osteoporosis. In fact, exercise has been shown to be an effective sexual enhancer as well as a bone protector.

Regular and consistent exercise not only is a good way to boost your mood but also can enhance your sex life and your relationship with your significant other. We often recommend that partners work out together when they can. Working out with your partner offers many advantages. First, if you know that you're working out with someone else, you are less likely to cancel or postpone your workout dates. Second, working out together promotes physical intimacy; it helps couples get back in synch with each other on a physical level, especially if they're having sexual difficulties. When couples haven't had sex in a while, it is often because one or both have gotten out of touch with their physical selves. There is often a disconnect with the physical aspects of life, not just in terms of sex but in paying attention to their bodies. Exercise is a great way to get partners to focus on their bodies in a positive way.

In the long run, regular exercise helps keep you slim and toned, which makes you feel good about your body. Studies suggest that fit people are more likely to feel they are desirable and to have more active sex lives than unfit people. This is as true for college students as for people old enough to be their parents. A 2000 study at Harvard University of 160 male and female swimmers in their 40s and 60s linked regular physical activity with more frequent and enjoyable sexual encounters.

Inspired to start working out? Turn to page 154.

## DO SOMETHING FOR YOURSELF

In the best of relationships, everyone needs some down time just for himself or herself. Having a hobby is a true mood booster that we encourage everyone to pursue. Carve out some time each week to pursue something that you love to do and that completely absorbs you, like playing a musical instrument, painting, needlepoint, sewing, making pottery, joining a softball league, bowling, playing pool, tai chi, Qigong, singing in a choir, or ballroom dancing (this is one you can do with your spouse). Your hobby should be something so engaging that it takes your mind off your daily concerns and allows you to truly enjoy yourself. If you feel guilty about taking time away from work or family, think of it this way: You will return to your responsibilities feeling refreshed, better able to perform at work and at a home.

## Staying Connected

A strong, satisfying relationship with your spouse or significant other is fundamental to your health and well-being. It's worth your time and effort to nurture your relationship.

Studies show that a good marriage dramatically enhances both physical health and emotional happiness, even more so for men than for women. Men fare better even in a bad marriage than living alone—married guys may *fantasize* about how much fun single life would be, but what they actually *need* is a stable, loving relationship with one person. The proof? Single guys are sicker, less happy, and die younger.

Women thrive in a happy marriage, but a not-so-good marriage can really take its toll, physically and emotionally. Nevertheless, long-term studies have taught us that with the exception of a violent marriage, couples who weather difficult times together end up happier—much happier—than couples who divorce. So it's important to take steps to maintain your marriage and a good mood, too.

Leisure activities—having fun together—are also vital to both personal happiness and successful relationships. This is where a couple can compensate for anything that might be missing in other realms of life. Your mood will be enhanced by having regular activities that take you away from work and the other stressors of life. It is important to recognize that leisure activities are vital to happy and successful lives.

However, this doesn't mean doing nothing. The kind of leisurely activity that promotes well-being is one that is highly engaging—whether it is a sport like tennis or golf, a pastime like gardening, or an artistic mode of expression like playing the piano together. In fact, having activities you both can be passionate about increases levels of positive emotion, vitality, and aliveness. In many cases these activities provide a sense of identity and social connection with other like-minded individuals, adding further to their positive impact. This aspect, paired with the known positive emotional and health impact of having a good marital relationship, makes active play with your life partner a winning combination.

# SELECTED BIBLIOGRAPHY

**CHAPTER ONE**
## WHEN SEX STOPS FEELING GOOD FOR HER

Meyer PM, Powel LH, Wilson RS, et al. A population-based longitudinal study of cognitive function in the menopausal transition. *Neurology* 2003; 61: 801–806.

Sex & Menopause Survey. www.redhotmamas.org/pdf/sex-newsletter/pdf.

Thompson RL. Menopause and brain function. *Neurology* 2003; 61: E9–E10.


**CHAPTER TWO**
## THE HARD TRUTH ABOUT SEX FOR HIM

Feldman HA, Goldstein DG, Hatzichristou RJ, et al. Impotence and its medical psychosocial correlates: results of the Massachusetts Male Aging Study. *J Urol* 1994; 151: 54–61.

Groessl EJ, Kaplan RM, Barrett-Connor E, et al. Overweight and obesity and the burden of disease and disability in elderly men. *Int J Obes Relat Metab Disord* 2004; 28: 1374–1382.

Johannes CB, Araujo HA, Feldman CA, et al. Incidence of erectile dysfunction in men 40 to 69 years old: longitudinal results from the Massachusetts male aging study. *J Urol* 2000; 163: 460–463.

Lindau SR, Schumm LP, Laumann EO, et al. A study of sexuality and health among older adults in the United States. *N Engl J Med* 2007; 357: 762–774.

Seidell JC, Bjorntorp P. Visceral fat accumulation in men positively associated with insulin, glucose and c-peptide levels, but negatively with testosterone. *Metabolism* 1990; 39: 897–901.

Selvin E, Burnett A, Platz E. Prevalence and risk factors for erectile dysfunction in the United States. *Am J Med* 2007; 120: 151–157.

Travison TG, Araujo AB, O'Donnell AB, et al. A population-level decline in serum testosterone levels in American men. *J Clin Endocrinol Metab* 2007; 92: 196–202.

### CHAPTER THREE
## WHEN YOU'RE FEELING DOWN

Heffner KL, Loving TJ, Kiecolt-Glaser JK. Older spouses'cortisol responses to marital conflict: associations with demand/withdraw communication patterns. *J Behav Med* 2006; 29: 317–325.

Kumano H. Osteoporosis and stress. *Clin Calcium* 2005; 9: 1544–1547.

Monti DM, Stoner M, et al. Complementary and Alternative Medicine. In Kornstein SG, Clayton AH (eds): *Women's Mental Health*. New York: Guilford, 2002, 344–356.

Sanchez O, Arnau A, Pareja M, et al. Acute stress-induced injury in mice: differences between emotional and social stress. *Cell Stress Chaperones* 2002; 7: 36–46.

van Gool CH, Kempen G, Penninx B, et al. Relationship between changes in depressive symptoms and unhealthy lifestyles in late middle aged and older persons: results from the Longitudinal Aging Study Amsterdam. *Age Ageing* 2003; 32: 81–87.

### CHAPTER FOUR
## THE LOWDOWN ON FAT

Arsenault BJ, Lachance D, Lemieux I, et al. Visceral adipose tissue accumulation, cardiorespiratory fitness and features of metabolic syndrome. *Arch Intern Med* 2007; 167: 1518–1525.

Kuo L, Kitlinska B, Tilan JU, et al. Neuropeptide Y acts directly in the periphery on fat tissue and mediates stress-induced obesity and metabolic syndrome.
*Nat Med* 2007; 13: 803—811.

Onat A, Avci GS, Barlan MM, et al. Measures of abdominal obesity assessed for visceral adiposity and relation to coronary risk. *Int J Obes Relat Metab Disord* 2004; 18: 1018–1025.

Rexrode KM, Carey VJ, Hennekens CH, et al. Abdominal obesity and coronary heart disease in women. *JAMA* 1998; 280: 1843–1848.

Rexrode KM, Buring JE, Manson JE. Abdominal and total adiposity and risk of coronary heart disease in men. *Int J Obes Relat Metab Disord* 2001; 25: 1047–1056.

Yan LL, Davidglus ML, Stamler J, et al. Midlife body mass index and hospitalization and mortaility in older age. *JAMA* 2006; 295; 190–198.

Yarnell JW, Patterson CC, Thomas HF, et al. Comparison of weight in middle age, weight at 18 years and weight change between, in predicting subsequent 14 year mortality and coronary events: Caerpilly Prospective Study. *J Epidemiol Community Health* 2000; 54: 344–348.

## CHAPTER FIVE
# NOT GETTING ANY SLEEP . . . FOR ALL THE WRONG REASONS

D'Souza A, Hassan S, Morgan D. Recent advances in surgery for snoring-somnplasty (radio-frequency palatoplasy) a pilot study: effectiveness and acceptability. *Rev Laryngol Otol Rhinol* 2000; 121: 111–115.

Grantved AM, Karup P. Complaints and satisfaction after uvulopalatopharyngoplasty. *Acta Otolaryngol Suppl* 2000; 543: 190–192.

Roosli C, Schneider S, Hausler R. Long term results and complications following uvulopala-topharyngoplasty in 116 consecutive patients. *Eur Arch Otorhinolaryngol* 2006; 263: 754–758.

Sleep in America Poll # 175, NSF 2005. www.sleepfoundation.org.

Sleep Apnea Information. American Sleep Apnea Association. www.sleepapnea.org.

Wilson C. A snorer's separate peace. *New York Times Home Magazine,* Spring 2007, 50–52.

## CHAPTER SIX
# SEX MAKEOVER

Basu A, Ryder RE. New treatment options for erectile dysfunction in patients with diabetes mellitus. *Drugs* 2004; 64: 2667–2688.

# SELECTED BIBLIOGRAPHY

Chetnik N. *VoiceMale: What Husbands Really Think About Their Marriages, Their Wives, Sex, Housework and Commitment.* New York: Simon & Schuster, 2006.

Meston CM, Gorzaika BB. The effects of sympathetic activation via acute exercise on physiological and subjective sexual arousal in women. *Behav Res Ther* 1995; 33: 651–664.

Schrobsdorff S. Price check in aisle sex. *Newsweek,* February 25, 2008, 15.

Sullivan O, Coltrane S. Men's changing contribution to housework and child care: a discussion paper on changing family roles. Prepared for the 11th Annual Conference of the Council on Contemporary Families, April 25–26, 2008, University of Illinois, Chicago.

## CHAPTER SEVEN
# DIET MAKEOVER

Campbell CT, Campbell TM II, Robbins J, et al. *The China Study: The Most Comprehensive Study of Nutrition Ever Conducted.* Dallas: Benbella Books, 2006.

Chos D, Badel S, Golav A. Micronutrition: a global approach for obese patients. *Rev Med Suisse* 2007; 3: 863–867.

Daubenmier J, Weidner G, Sumner M, et al. The contribution of changes in diet, exercise and stress management to changes in coronary risk in women and men in multisite cardiac lifestyle intervention program. *Ann Behav Med* 2007; 33: 57–68.

Ferguson LR, Philpott M. Cancer prevention by dietary bioactive components that target the immune response. *Cur Cancer Drug Targets* 2007; 7: 459–464.

Hanninen O, Rauma AL, Kaartinen K, et al. Vegan diet in physiological health promotion. *Acta Physiol Hung* 1999; 86: 171–180.

Hu FB, Willett WC. Optimal diets for prevention of coronary heart disease. *JAMA* 2002; 288: 2569–2578.

Johns JH, Ziebland S, Yudkin P, et al. Effects of fruits and vegetable consumption on plasma antioxidant concentrations and blood pressure: a randomized controlled trial. *Lancet* 2002; 359: 1969–1974.

Lampe JW. Spicing up a vegetarian diet: chemoprotective effects of phytochemicals. *Am J Clin Nutr* 2003; 78 (suppl): 579S–583S.

Steck SE, Gaudet MM, Eng SM, et al. Cooked meat and risk of breast cancer: lifetime versus recent dietary intake. *Epidemiology* 2007; 18: 373–382.

**CHAPTER EIGHT**
# EXERCISE MAKEOVER

Bacon CG, Mittleman MA, Kawachi I, et al. Sexual function in men older than 50 years of age: results the health professionals follow-up study. *Ann Intern Med* 2003; 139: 161–168.

Penhollow TM, Younger M. Sexual desirability and sexual performance: does exercise and fitness really matter? *Electronic Journal of Human Sexuality* 2004; 7: October 5.

Puetz TW, O'Connor PJ, Dishman RK. Effects of chronic exercise on feelings of energy and fatigue: a quantitative synthesis. *Psychol Bull* 2006; 132: 866–876.


**CHAPTER NINE**
# HORMONE MAKEOVER

Bolona ER, Uraga MV, Haddad RM, et al. Testosterone use in men with sexual dysfunction: a systematic review and meta-analysis of randomized placebo-controlled trials. *Mayo Clin Proc* 2007; 82: 20–28.

Basso R, Schultz WW. Sexual sequelae of general medical disorders. *Lancet* 2007; 369: 409–424.

Bren L. The estrogen and progestin dilemma: new advice, labeling guidelines. U.S. Food and Drug Administration, *FDA Consumer Magazin,* 2003; 37: 10–11.

Cavalieri E, Rogan E. Catechol quinones of estrogens in the initiation of breast, prostate, and other human cancers. *Ann NY Acad Sci* 2006; 1089: 286–301.

Rohan TE, Negassa A, Chlebowski, RT, et al. Conjugated equine estrogen and risk of benign proliferative breast disease: a randomized controlled trial. *J Natl Cancer Inst* 2008; 100: 563–571.

David SR, Walker KZ, Strauss BJ. Effects of estradiol with and without testosterone on body composition and relationships with lipids in postmenopausal women. *Menopause* 2000; 7: 395–401.

Heiss G, Wallace R, Anderson GL, et al. for the WHI Investigators. Health risks and benefits 3 years after stopping randomized treatment with estrogen and progestin. JAMA 2008; 299: 1036–1045.

Hulley B, Grady D. The WHI estrogen-alone trial: do things look any better? *JAMA* 2004; 291: 1673.

Langer RD. Progestins: pharmacologic characteristics and clinically relevant differences. *Int J Fertil* 2000: 45 (suppl 1): 63–72.

Manson JE, Allison MA, Roussouw JE, et al. Estrogen therapy and coronary-artery calcification. *N Engl J Med* 2007; 356: 2591–2602.

Natrajan PK, Soumakis K, Gambrell RD Jr. Estrogen replacement therapy in women with previous breast cancer. *Am J Obstet Gynecol* 1999; 181: 288–295.

Savvas M. Increase in bone mass after one year of percutaneous oestradiol and testosterone implants in postmenopausal women who have previously received long-term oral oestrogens. *Br J Obstet Gynaecol* 1992; 99: 757–760.

Seed M, Sands RH, McLaren M, et al. The effect of hormone replacement therapy and route of administration on selected cardiovascular risk factors in postmenopausal women. *Fam Pract* 2000; 17: 497–507.

Studd J, Magos A. Hormone pellet implantation for the menopause and premenstrual syndrome. *Obstet Gynecol Clin North Am* 1987; 14: 229–249.

Wang C, Cunningham G, Dobs A, et al. Long-term testosterone gel (Androgel) treatment maintains beneficial effects on sexual function and mood, lean and fat mass, and bone mineral density in hypogonadal men. *Clin Endocrinol Metab* 2004; 89: 2085–2098.

Wilson, Robert. *Forever Female.* New York: M. Evans & Co., 1968.

Women's Health Initiative Estrogen plus progestin study stopped due to increased breast cancer risk, lack of overall benefit.

Wright, J. Bio-identical steroid hormone replacement: selected observations from 23 years of clinical and laboratory practice. *Ann NY Acad Sci* 2005; 1057: 506–524.

## CHAPTER TEN
# SUPPLEMENT MAKEOVER

Alba-Roth J, Muler OA, Schopohl J, et al. Arginine stimulates growth hormone secretion by suppressing endogenous somatostatin secretion. *J Clin Endocrin Metab* 1988; 67: 1186–1189.

Birch R, Noble D, Greenhaff PL. The influence of dietary creatine supplementation on performance during repeated bouts of maximal isokinetic cycling in man. *Eur J Appl Physiol* 1994; 69: 268–270, 1994.

Brass EP, Hiatt WR. The role of carnitine and carnitine supplementation during exercise in man and in individuals with special needs. *J Am Coll Nutr* 1998; 17: 207–215.

Casey A, Constantin-Teodosiu D, Howell S, et al. Creatine ingestion favorably affects perfor-mance and muscle metabolism during maximal exercise in humans. *Am J Physiol* 1996; 34: E31–37.

Colombani P, Wenk C, Kunz I, et al. Effects of L-carnitine supplementation on physical per-formance and energy metabolism of endurance-trained athletes: a double-blind crossover field study. *Eur J Appl Physiol Occup Physiol* 1996; 73: 434–439.

Harris RC, Soderlund K, Hultman E. Elevation of creatine in resting and exercised muscle of normal subjects by creatine supplementation. *Clin Sci (Lond)* 1992; 83: 367–374.

Jang M, Cai L, Odeani G, et al. Cancer chemopreventive activity of resveratrol, a natural product derived from grapes. *Science* 1997; 275: 218–220.

Liong, MT. Probiotics: a critical review of their potential role as antihypertensives, immune modulators, hypocholesterolemics, and perimenopausal treatments. *Nutr Rev* 2007; 65: 316–328.

National Cancer Institute. Calcium glucarate. NCI drug dictionary. www.cancer,gov/ Templates/drugdictionary.

National Center for Complementary and Alternative Medicine and Office of Dietary Supple-ments. Questions and answers on the safety of black cohosh and the symptoms of meno-pause. 2005; http://nccam.nih.gov/health.

Simopoulos AP. Omega-3 fatty acids and athletes. *Curr Sports Med Rep* 2007; 6: 230–236.

Sinclair AJ, Begg D, Mathai M, et al. Omega-3 fatty acids and the brain: a review of studies in depression. *Asia Pac J Clin Nutr* 2007; 16 (Suppl 1): 391–397.

Soop M. Influence of carnitine supplementation on muscle substrate and carnitine metabo-lism during exercise. *J Appl Physiol* 1988; 2394–2399.

Trappe SW, Costill DL, Goodpaster B, et al. The effects of L-carnitine supplementation on performance during interval swimming. *Int J Sports Med* 1994; 15: 181–185.

**CHAPTER ELEVEN**

# MOOD MAKEOVER

Bensen, Herbert. *The Relaxation Response.* New York: Avon Books, 1976.

Blumenthal JA, Babyak MA, Moore KA, et al. Effects of exercise training on older patients with major depression. *Arch Intern Med* 1999; 159: 2349–2356.

## SELECTED BIBLIOGRAPHY

Brown RP, Gerbarg PL. Sudarshan Kriya Yogic breathing in the treatment of stress, anxiety, and depression. Part II—clinical applications and guidelines. *J Altern Complement Med* 2001; 11: 711–717. Haney E, Chan B, Diem S, et al, for the Osteoporotic Fractures in Men Study Group. Association of low bone mineral density with selective serotonin re-uptake inhibitor use by older men. *Arch Intern Med* 2007; 167: 1246–1251.

# INDEX

Abdominal aortic aneurysm, screening for, 205
Accupril (quinapril), 15, 31
ACE inhibitors, 15
   sexual dysfunction and, 31
Affection, nonsexual, 16
Age
   menopause and, 6
   probiotics and, 212
   stress and, 43
AIDS, 106
Alcohol
   sexual dysfunction and, 28
   snoring and, 73
Aldactone (Spironolactone), 32
Aldosterone antagonist, 32
Alpha-inhibitors, 15
   sexual dysfunction and, 31
Alprostadil, 105
Altace (ramipril), 15, 31
Ambien, 82–83
*American Journal of Clinical Nutrition,* 216
*American Journal of Medicine,* 30
*American Journal of Preventive Medicine,* 124
Amitriptyline (Elavil), 15, 31
AndroGel, 19, 186
Andropause, ix
Animal fat, 124–125
Antidepressants, viii
   sexual dysfunction and, 31
   for women, 14–15
Antihistamines, 66
   snoring and, 73
Antihypertensives
   to lower blood pressure, 31
   sexual dysfunction and, 31
   for women, 15
Antioxidants, 43, 132
Anxiety, 36
Aphrodisiacs, 113
   herbal, 226–227, 228
*Archives of Internal Medicine,* 237
Arginine, 225
Atenolol (Tenormin), 15, 31

Atorvastatin (Lipitor), 32
Autoimmune disease, in women, 9
Autonomic nervous system, 39
Ayurvedic medicine, 225

*B. bifidum,* 211
Back exercise, 168–169
Bed
   elevation, 74
   sheets and, 80
   sleep and, 69–80
Benazepril (Lotensin), 15, 31
Benign prostate hypertrophy (BPH), 202
Benson-Henry Institute of Mind-Body Medicine, 231
Benzodiazepines, 81
Beta-blockers, viii, 15
   sexual dysfunction and, 31
BHRT. *See* Bioequivalent hormones
Biceps exercise, 170–171
Binging, 131
Bioequivalent hormones (BHRT), 177, 180, 185–186
   common brands, 199–200
   dose, 198
   pharmaceutical goals, 194
Black cohosh *(Cimicifuga racemosa),* 227
Blood sugar. *See also* Diabetes
   abnormal levels of, 25
BMI. *See* Body mass index
Body mass index (BMI), 26
   calculating, 53
   snoring and, 76
   waist-to-hip ratio, 52–53
Bones, 10. *See also* Osteoporosis
Bone scan, 189, 205
BPH. *See* Benign prostate hypertrophy
Brain, stress and, 43
Breakfast, 142–144
Breast cancer, screening, 188
Breathing, 230–232
*British Journal of Nutrition,* 131
Bruxism, 70

Calan (verapamil), 15, 32
Calcium, 128
Calcium channel blockers, 15
   sexual dysfunction and, 32
Calcium-D-glucarate, 99, 221–222
   dose, 221
Calf stretching, 162–164
Campbell, Dr. T. Colin, 128–129
Cancer, screening, 188, 204
Capoten (captopril), 15, 31
Capsaicin, 131–132
Captopril (Capoten), 15, 31
Carbohydrates, recommended, 148
Cardizem (diltiazem), 15, 32
Cardura (doxazosin), 15, 31
Carnitine, 214–216
   dose, 214
Carvedilol (Coreg), 15, 31
Caverject (prostaglandin E1), 105
Cervical cancer, screening, 188
Chamomile, 81
Cheese, 139
Chest exercises, 169–170, 233
*The China Study* (Campbell), 128–129
Chinese medicine, 225
Chlorothiazide (Diuril), 32
Cholesterol, 54–56
   triglycerides and, 55–56
   types of, 54
Cholesterol lowering drugs, sexual dysfunction
   and, 32
Cialis (tadalafil), xii, 17, 101, 104
Cimetidine (Tagamet), 15, 32
*Cimicifuga racemosa* (Black cohosh), 227
Circulation, in men, 21
Coenzyme Q10 (CoQ10), 217
   dose, 217
Cognition, in women during menopause, 11
Colonoscopy, 188, 204
Communication, 113–119
   mood booster for couples, 235
Condoms, 106, 107
Continuous positive airway pressure (CPAP)
   device, 78
Cooking, 62–63
Coreg (carvedilol), 15, 31
Core rotation exercise, 174–175
Coumadin, 214
Counseling, 114
   marriage, 47
CPAP. *See* Continuous positive airway pressure
   device
Cravings, 145
C-reactive protein, 25, 57
Creatine, 218–219
   dose, 218
Crestor (rosuvastatin), 32

Dalmane, 81
Damiana, 228
Depression
   heart disease and, 44
   in men, 237–238
DEXA bone density test, 188–189, 205
DHA. *See* Docosahexaenoic acid
DHT. *See* Dihydrotestosterone
Diabetes
   ethnicity and, 60
   excess body fat and, 52
   heart disease and, 59
   prediabetes, 19–20
   resveratrol and, 224
   screening, 188, 204
   sex and, 59
   sexual problems with, 14
   type 1, 57–58
   type 2, 58–59, 134–135
Diet
   binging, 131
   guidelines, 136
   healthful, 47–48
   inflammatory factors and, 25
   kitchen preparation, 140–141
   lifestyle makeover, xiv
   meal planning, 142–149
   sabotaging, 153
   vegetables, 136–137
Diet makeover, 122–153
   better food choices for better sex, 123–127
   with partner, 123
Digital rectal exam (DRE), 204
Dihydrotestosterone (DHT), 23, 191, 206
Diindoyl-methane (DIM), 99, 222–223
   dose, 222
Dilaudid (hydromorphone), 15, 32
Diltiazem (Cardizem), 15, 32
DIM. *See* Diindoyl-methane
Dinner, 144–145
Diuretics, 219
   sexual dysfunction and, 32
Diuril (chlorothiazide), 32
Docosahexaenoic acid (DHA), 213
Doxazosin (Cardura), 15, 31
DRE. *See* Digital rectal exam
Drugs. *See also* individual drug names
   over-the-counter, 75
   sex-busting, for women, 14–15
   sexual dysfunction and, 29
   side effects, 29
   for treatment of erectile dysfunction, 100–104
Dyslipidemia, 25

*E. Coli,* 133–134
ED. *See* Erectile dysfunction
Effexor (venlafaxine), 31

Eicosapentaenoic acid (EPA), 213
Elavil (amitriptyline), 15, 31
Emotions, 109–111
Enalapril (Vasotec), 15, 31
Endorphins, 28, 113
Enteric nervous system, 39
Enzymes, 101
EPA. *See* Eicosapentaenoic acid
*Epimedium* extract, 226
Erectile dysfunction (ED), vii, 16–32
    animal fat and, 125
    causes, 20–25
    definition, 16–17
    medications for, xii–xiii
    performance anxiety, 28
    treatment with penile implants, 105
    treatment with penile injections, 105
    treatment with prescription drugs,
        100–104
Escitalopram (Lexapro), 31
Estradiol, 7, 190, 196, 205
Estriol, 7
Estrogen, 7–8, 181
    in men, 23–24
    during menopause, 5
    role in learning and memory, 10
    screening, 192–193
    supplements, 220–224
    types of, 7
    weight gain and, 50
Estrone, 7, 190
Ethnicity, diabetes and, 60
Eucalyptus oil, 73
*European Heart Journal,* 20
Exercise
    as an aphrodisiac, 113
    lifestyle makeover, xiv
    relationships and, 63
    sexual dysfunction and, 30
    snoring and, 75
Exercise makeover, 154–176
    back, 168–169
    biceps, 170–171
    chest, 169–170
    core rotation, 174–175
    front stabilization, 175–176
    hips and glutes, 172–174
    overview, 154–156
    shoulders, 166–167
    squats, 165
    stretching, 156–164
    triceps, 171–172

Fat, 141
    abdominal, 51–53
    animal, 124–125
    diabetes and, 52

epidemic, 48–51
    inflammation and, 56–57
    mono-unsaturated, 127
    trans, 51–52, 125–127
    weight and, 46–63
Felodipine (Plendil), 15, 32
*Feminine Forever* (Wilson), 181
Fenofibrate (Tricor), 32
Fentanyl (Fentora), 15, 32
Fentora (fentanyl), 15, 32
Fibrates, sexual dysfunction and, 32
Fish, 138
Flavonoids, 132
Flaxseeds, 141, 214
Fluoxetine (Prozac), 14, 31
Fluvoxamine (Luvox), 82
Follicle-stimulating hormone (FSH), 6–7, 22, 189,
        205
Food
    plant-based, 131–135
    recommended, 148–149
    serving size, 147
    snoring and, 75
    unprocessed, 130
Free radicals, 43
Front stabilization exercise, 175–176
Fruit
    recommended, 149
    serving size, 149
FSH. *See* Follicle-stimulating hormone

GABA. *See* Gamma-aminobutyric acid
Gamma-aminobutyric acid (GABA), 81
Gemfibrozil (Lopid), 32
Geriatricians, ix–x
Gonorrhea, 106
Gotu kola (*Centella asiatica*), 81
Grains, 133, 139–140. *See also* Protein
    recommended, 149
"G" spot, 108
Gynecomastia, 202

Halcion, 81
Hamstring stretch, 157–160
$H_2$ antagonists, 15
    sexual dysfunction and, 32
Harvard Nurses' Health Study, 128
HDL. *See* High-density lipoprotein
Heart, stress and, 43–44
Heart disease, 43–44
    death from, 59
    diabetes and, 59
Heart/Estrogen Progestin Replacement Study
        (HERS Study), 183–184
Heavy metal toxicity, 25–26
Hemp seed protein, 219–220
    dose, 219

Herbs
  as aphrodisiacs, 226–227, 228
  for sleep, 81
HERS Study (Heart/Estrogen Progestin
    Replacement Study), 183–184
High-density lipoprotein (HDL), 54–55
Hips and glutes exercise, 172–174, 233
HIV infection, 106
Hops, 81
Hormone makeover, 177–208. *See also* Hormone
    replacement therapy; Hormones
  for men, 201–208
  options, 193–200, 206–208
  overview, 177–179
  for women, 179–200
Hormone replacement therapy (HRT), xi, 177.
    *See also* Hormone makeover; Hormones;
    Menopause
  history, 181–182
  for men, 98
  for symptoms caused by menopause,
    4–5
  for women, 106
Hormones. *See also* Hormone makeover;
    Hormone replacement therapy;
    Metabolism
  creams and gels, 195–196
  levels of, 22
  lifestyle makeover, xiv
  in men, 98–99
  pellets, 197, 208
  pills, 194–195
  rebalancing, xi–xiii
  screening, 189
  sleep and, 67
Hot flashes, 4
HRT. *See* Hormone replacement therapy
Hunger, 131
Hydromorphone (Dilaudid), 15, 32
Hyperthyroidism, 24
Hypothyroidism, 24–25

IL–6, 25
Immune system
  probiotics and, 212
  stress and, 44
Inderal (propranolol), 15, 31
Indian medicine, 225
Indole-3-carbinol, 99, 222
Inflammation, 25
  fat and, 56–57
Insomnia, 4, 69–70. *See also* Sleep
  sexual dysfunction and, 29
  short-term, 69
Insulin levels, 19
Integrative medicine, x
Intimacy, 119–121

*Journal of Clinical Endocrinology and Metabolism,*
    202
*Journal of the National Cancer Institute,* 184

Kabat-Zinn, Jon, 236
Kama Sutra, 111
KFC, 126
Klonopin (Clonazepam), 81

*Lactobacillus acidophilus,* 211
*Lactobacillus bulgaricus,* 211
*The Lancet,* 68
Latissimus stretching, 161–162
LDL. *See* Low-density lipoprotein
Leisure activities, 239
Lexapro (escitalopram), 31
Levitra (vardenafil), xii, 17, 101
LH. *See* Luteinizing hormone
Libido, viii, xvi. *See also* Erectile
    dysfunction
  in women, 3–15
Lifestyle. *See also* Diabetes
  changes in, xi
  during menopause, 14
  skin changes and, 9
  snoring and, 72–75
Lipitor (atorvastatin), 32
Lopid (gemfibrozil), 32
Lopressor (metoprolol), 15, 31
Lotensin (benazepril), 15, 31
Lovastatin (Mevacor), 32
Low-density lipoprotein (LDL), 54–55
LP-PLA2, 25
Lubricants, 107
Lunch, 144–145
Lunesta (eszopiclone), 83
Luteinizing hormone (LH), 7, 22

Maca (*Lepidium meyenii*), 227
Magnesium, 81
Manerix (moclobemide), 31
MAOIs, sexual dysfunction and, 31
Marriage, 239–240. *See also* Relationships
  counseling, 47
  stress and, 38–39
  weight gain and, 46–47
Massachusetts Male Aging Study, 16, 26
Massage oil, 108
MBSR. *See* Mindfulness-based stress reduction
McDonald's, 126
Meal planning, 142–149
  breakfast, 142–144
  lunch/dinner, 144–145
  menus, 150–152
  serving size, 147
  snacks, 144
Meditation, 231

Melatonin, 67
  supplements for sleep, 81
Memory, during menopause, 10–11
Men. *See also* Erectile dysfunction
  animal fat and, 125
  circulation in, 21
  hormone makeover, 201–208
  hormones and, 98–99
  nerve damage and, 21
  prediabetes and, 19–20
  preventive health exam, 204–208
  sex drive in, 12
  sexual dysfunction in, 16–32
  sexual health, 89, 90–91
  sexual makeover, 97–100
  stress in, 37–38
  weight gain and, 50–51
Menopause, vii. *See also* Hormone replacement
    therapy
  age and, 6
  bone and muscle, 10
  description, 6–11
  hormonal ups and downs, 7–8
  hormones during, 5
  memory and mood, 10–11
  osteoporosis and, 10
  resveratrol and, 224
  sex after, 3–4
  skin changes, 9
  vaginal thinning, 9
  vulnerable periods during, 8
  weight gain and, 49–50
Menstruation, 6–7
Menus, 150–152
Metabolic syndrome, 19–20. *See also* Diabetes
Metabolism, 22–23. *See also* Hormones
  during sleep, 68
Metoprolol (Lopressor), 15, 31
Metoprolol succinate (Toprol XL), 15, 31
Mevacor (lovastatin), 32
Midlife
  changes in, ix
  crises, xvii–ix
  fat and, 48–51
  physical changes during, 17
  transition to, 5
Mindfulness-based stress reduction (MBSR),
    236–237
Minipress (prazosin), 15, 31
Moclobemide (Manerix), 31
Mono-unsaturated fat, 127
Mood makeover, 229–240
  breathing, 230–232
  exercise, 237–238
  finding joy in life, 234–235
  mindfulness-based stress reduction, 236–237
  muscle awareness, 233–234

  overview, 229–230
  relationships, 235
  something for yourself, 238–240
  stretching, 232–233
Moods, 35–45, 90
  capsaicin and, 131–132
  lifestyle makeover, xv
  during menopause, 10–11
  sexual makeover and, 93–94
  sleep and, 78–81
  stress and, viii
  swings, 4
Muira puama *(Ptychopetalum olacoides),*
    226–228
Multivitamins, 37, 210–211
Muscles, 10
  awareness, 233–234
Music, sleep and, 779

Nardil (phenelzine), 31
National Center for Complementary and
    Alternative Medicine (NCCAM), 227
National Institutes of Health (NIH), 126, 182, 218
National Sleep Association, 64
National Sleep Foundation, 65
NCCAM. *See* National Center for
    Complementary and Alternative Medicine
*New England Journal of Medicine,* 18
*New York Times,* 80
Nifedipine (Procardia), 15, 32
NIH. *See* National Institutes of Health
Nitric oxide (NO), 101
NO. *See* Nitric oxide
Non-rapid eye movement (NREM) activity, 66
Nortriptyline (Pamelor), 31
NREM. *See* Non-rapid eye movement activity
NSAIDs, 66
Nuts, 132–133, 141
  recommended, 149

Obesity. *See also* Weight
  stress and, 42
Oils, 133, 141
Omega-3 fatty acids, 25, 212–214
  cautions, 214
  dose, 212
Omega-6 fatty acids, 213
Omega-3 fatty acid supplements, 25, 37
Opioids, 15
  sexual dysfunction and, 32
Orgasms, viii
  achievement of, 13–14
  delays in, 13–14
Osteoporosis
  menopause and, 10
  screening, 188–189
Oxycodone (Percodan), 15, 32

PAI-1, 25
Painkillers, 15
  sexual dysfunction and, 32
  for women, 15
Pamelor (nortriptyline), 31
Papaverine hydrochloride, 105
Parasympathetic nervous system, 39
Paroxetine (Paxil), 14, 31
Passion flower, 81
Patients
  history, 22
  physical, examination 22–25
Paxil (paroxetine), 14, 31
PDE5. *See* Phosphodiesterase type 5
Pectoral stretch, 160–161
Penile implants, 105
Penile injections, 105
Percodan (oxycodone), 15, 32
Performance anxiety, in men, 28
Phenelzine (Nardil), 31
Phentolamine (Regitine), 105
Phosphodiesterase type 5 (PDE5), 101
Physical examination, 22–25, 203–208
  for men, 203–208
  preventive, 187–192
  for women, 187
Physicians
  lifestyle makeover and, xv–xvi
  men's relationship with, 18
Phytochemicals, 43
Phytoestrogens, 139
Plendil (felodipine), 15, 32
*Polygonum cuspidatum* (resveratrol), 223–224
Polymorphisms, 210–211
Polyphenols, 132
Polyunsaturated fatty acids (PUFAs), 126–127
Prazosin (Minipress), 15, 31
Premarin, 182, 184
PREMPRO, 182
Probiotics, 211–212
Procardia (nifedipine), 15, 32
Progesterone, 7, 191
  during menopause, 5
  sleep and, 67
Progestin, 181–182
Propranolol (Inderal), 15, 31
Prostaglandin E1 (Caverject), 105
Prostate cancer, screening, 204–205
Prostate-specific antigen (PSA) test, 204
Protein, 123. *See also* Grains
  animal-based versus plant-based, 127–128, 138
  dairy, 128
  hemp seed, 219–220
  lean, 137–139
  recommended, 148
Prozac (fluoxetine), 14, 31

PSA. *See* Prostate-specific antigen test
*Ptychopetalum olacoides* (Muira puama)
  for men, 226–227
  for women, 227–228
Puberty, 23
PUFAs. *See* Polyunsaturated fatty acids
Puncturevine *(Tribulus terrestris),* 225–226

Quinapril (Accupril), 15, 31
Quinoa, 133

Ramipril (Altace), 15, 31
Ranitidine (Zantac), 15, 32
Rapid eye movement (REM), 66
Recipes
  Anthony's simple sprout salad, 146–147
  Dan's easy dressing, 146
  Dan's easy salad, 146
  Dan's trail mix, 145–146
  Presto pesto, 147
Red peppers, 131
Regitine (phentolamine), 105
Relationships, 29–30, 44–45, 90. *See also* Marriage
  cooking, 62–63
  exercise, 63
  mood booster, 235
  sexual makeover and, 95–97
  shopping, 61–62
  weight gain and, 61–63
Relaxation techniques, 37
REM. *See* Rapid eye movement
Restless legs syndrome (RLS), 69–70
Resveratrol, 223–224
  dose, 223
Rice, 140
RLS. *See* Restless legs syndrome
Rosemary (herb), 132
Rosuvastatin (Crestor), 32
Rozerem (Ramelteon), 82

Seeds, 141
  recommended, 149
Serotonin inhibitors, sexual dysfunction and, 31
Sertraline (Zoloft), 14, 31
Sex
  after menopause, 3–4
  decline in, viii
  diabetes and, 59
  emotions and, 109–111
  foreplay and, 108
  lack of interest in, 88
  lifestyle makeover, xiii–xiv
  men and, 16–32
  positions, 108–109
  safe, 106